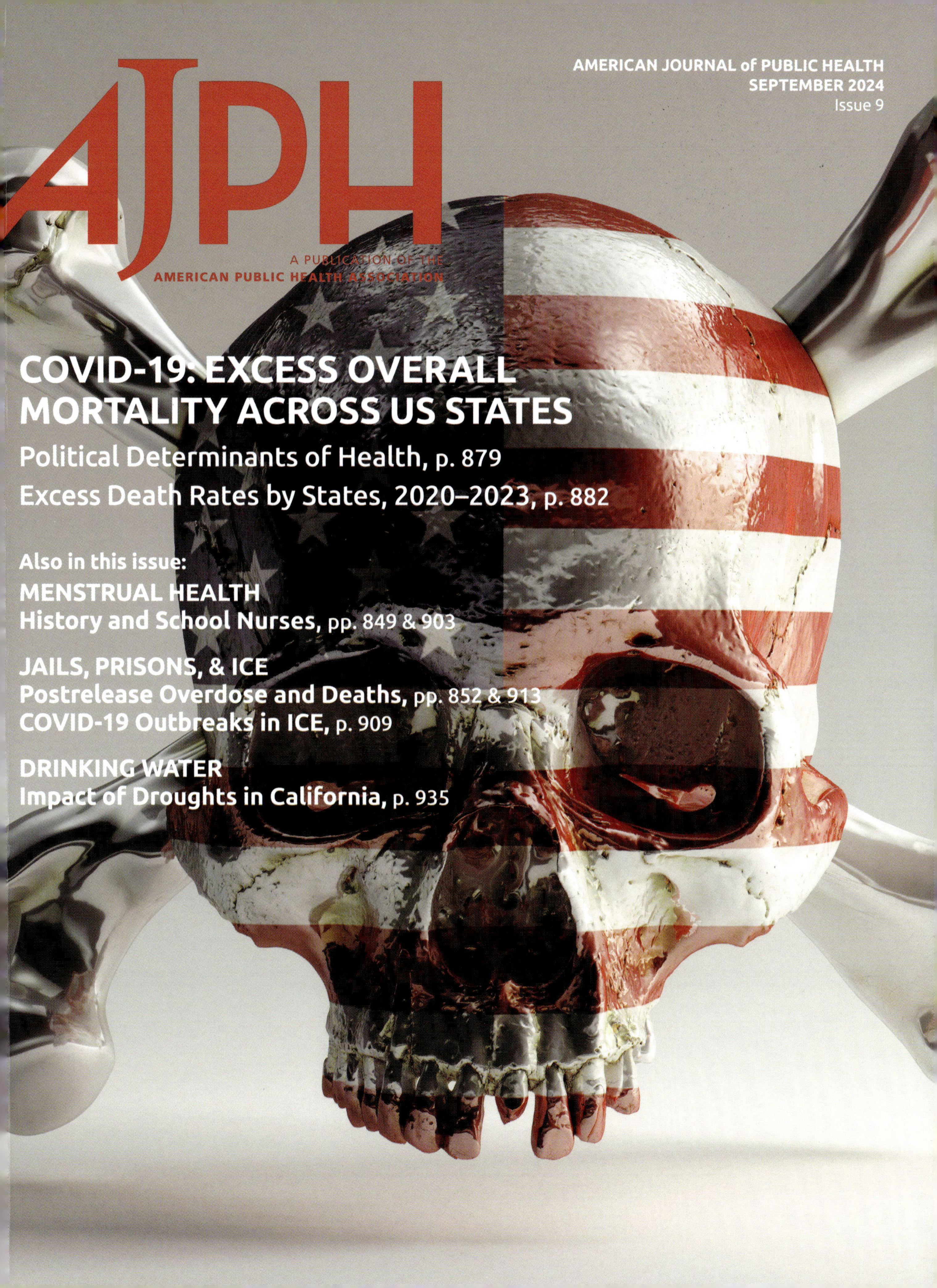

AMERICAN JOURNAL of PUBLIC HEALTH
SEPTEMBER 2024
Issue 9

AJPH

A PUBLICATION OF THE
AMERICAN PUBLIC HEALTH ASSOCIATION

COVID-19: EXCESS OVERALL MORTALITY ACROSS US STATES

Political Determinants of Health, p. 879
Excess Death Rates by States, 2020–2023, p. 882

Also in this issue:

MENSTRUAL HEALTH
History and School Nurses, pp. 849 & 903

JAILS, PRISONS, & ICE
Postrelease Overdose and Deaths, pp. 852 & 913
COVID-19 Outbreaks in ICE, p. 909

DRINKING WATER
Impact of Droughts in California, p. 935

APHA
AMERICAN PUBLIC HEALTH ASSOCIATION
For science. For action. For health.

AJPH®, published monthly, is the official Journal of the American Public Health Association®, 800 I St NW, Washington, DC 20001-3710; (202) 777- APHA; TDD (202) 777-2500. APHA is a nongovernmental professional society founded in 1872, representing all disciplines and specialties in public health.

The *American Journal of Public Health*® (*AJPH*) (print ISSN: 0090-0036; electronic ISSN: 1541- 0048), first published in 1911, is the official journal of the American Public Health Association® (APHA). The oldest and largest organization of public health professionals in the world, APHA represents approximately 30 000 members from more than 50 occupations of public health.

Submissions: Visit www.editorialmanager.com/ajph or ajph.edmgr.com for online manuscript preparation and submission guidelines. Contributions of original unpublished research, social science analyses, scholarly essays, critical commentaries, departments, and letters to the editor are welcome. Questions? Write ajph.submissions@apha.org or call APHA at (202) 777-2469.

Print plus online subscriptions: Institutional price (print copy with online access for a single institution and all authorized users, regardless of geographic location) varies by size of organization and ranges from $993–$1445 for US organizations, and $1073–$1526 for international organizations (air delivery); multiple campuses not permitted without special arrangement. Details of the tiered pricing system at https://subscriptionoffice.com/pages/apha-landing-page. To order, write apha.subscriptions@apha.org.

Online-only subscriptions: Institutional price for one institution and its authorized users (regardless of geographic location) is $878–$1307. To order, write apha.subscriptions@apha.org. For academic consortia or multisite corporate subscriptions, contact apha.subscriptions@apha.org.

Print-only subscriptions: Institutional price is US $701, $782 international.

Back print issues: A limited number of print issues are for sale. Single copies are US $49, $55 international (air delivery). Shipping included; prepay only. To order, write apha.subscriptions@apha.org.

Reprints: For prices and ordering information on 50 or more reprints, check the Reprints section at www.ajph.org. To order smaller quantities of reprints (rush delivery), use the "Purchase Article" link on the article site itself.

Electronic access: Online articles more than 10 years old are available free for personal use at www.ajph.org. Recent articles are available through pay-per-view: single PDF article for $24, single issue access for 24 hours for $33, or entire site access for 24 hours for $38.

Postal information: Periodicals postage paid at Washington, DC, and additional mailing offices. Postmaster: Send address changes to American Journal of Public Health, 800 I St NW, Washington, DC 20001-3710.

Address changes: Send to AJPH, Membership Department (members) or AJPH Subscriptions (subscribers), APHA, 800 I St NW, Washington, DC 20001-3710. Or write to membership.mail@apha. org (members) or apha.subscriptions@apha.org (subscribers).

Advertising: For pricing and other information, see www.ajph.org. Please write to ashell.alston@apha.org or call (202) 777-2470 for other advertising opportunities. Ask about special exhibit packages and sponsorships. Acceptance of advertising by the *Journal* does not imply endorsement of products.

Indexes: Publications that index or abstract articles from *AJPH* include the following: Ageline, Assia (Applied Social Science Index and Abstracts), Biological Abstracts, Chemical Abstracts, CINAHL, Criminal Justice Abstracts, EMBASE, EMCare, Environmental Abstracts, e-psyche, ERIC, ETOH (Alcohol and Alcohol Problems Science Database), Excerpta Medica, Food Science and Technology, General Science Index, Grateful Med, Hospital Literature Index, Human Resources Abstracts, International Pharmaceutical Abstracts (IPA), Medline, Physical Education Index, Pollution Abstracts, Psychological Abstracts, PsychINFO, Safety Science Abstracts, Sage Family Studies Abstracts, Sage Human Resources Abstracts, Science Citation Index, SCOPUS, SIIC Data Bases, Social Work Research and Abstracts, and Statistical Reference Index (SRI)/LexisNexis.

Medscape Publishers' Circle

AJPH

A PUBLICATION OF THE
AMERICAN PUBLIC HEALTH ASSOCIATION

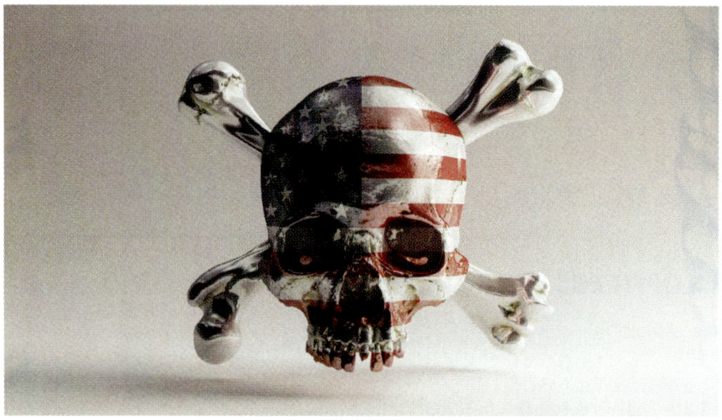

COVER: As the COVID-19 pandemic unfolded, the rate of excess deaths varied across the 50 US states and was associated with the partisan orientation of governors and state legislatures.

Cover concept and selection by Aleisha Kropf. Image by Paul Campbell/iStock. Printed with permission.

APHA
AMERICAN PUBLIC HEALTH ASSOCIATION
For science. For action. For health.

Promoting public health research, policy, practice, and education is the *AJPH* mission. As we widen our scope to embrace global issues, we also sharpen our focus to support the needs of public health practitioners. We invite contributions of original unpublished research, opinion and commentary, and letters to the editor.

The *Journal* is printed on acid-free recycled paper.

OPEN ACCESS ONLINE ONLY PODCAST DATA SUPPLEMENT AVAILABLE

EDITOR'S CHOICE

844 The Next Generation of LGBTQ+ Health in *AJPH*
B. E. Coston and S. Landers

BOOKS & MEDIA

846 Advancing, Prioritizing, and Uplifting Equitable Strategies to Improve Black Women's Reproductive Health and Sexuality Wellness
T. C. Willie

OPINIONS, IDEAS, & PRACTICE

EDITORIALS

849 School Nurses and the Promotion of Inclusive Menstrual Health
D. Tobbell

852 Know the Difference Between Jail and Prison? Both Are Associated With Risk of Death
J. Berk and L. Brinkley-Rubinstein

856 Mass Incarceration and Health Inequities: A Public Health of Consequence, September 2024
F. Kapadia

PERSPECTIVES

859 Optimizing Wastewater Surveillance: The Necessity of Standardized Reporting and Proficiency for Public Health
I. Keenum, N. J. Lin, A. Logan-Jackson, A. J. Gushgari, N. D'Souza, J. A. Steele, D. Kaya, and L. R. Gushgari

864 Educational Outcomes Are an Underused Metric for Child and Life Course Health
N. L. Sprague, C. C. Branas, A. G. Rundle, and P. Factor-Litvak

NOTES FROM THE FIELD

870 Building Power on "Mass&Cass": A Community-Centered Approach to Addressing Health Resource Gaps for Persons Experiencing Homelessness in Boston, MA, 2021
K. I. King Jr, E. Milien, M. Jones, T. Mensah, and L. L. E. J. Carty

874 Scaling Emergency Department Opioid Use Disorder Treatment Across California to Reduce Overdose Deaths, 2019–2023
E. A. Samuels, A. D. Rosen, M. Speener, J. Kaleekal, M. M. Kalmin, D. Goodman-Meza, S. Shoptaw, S. Clayton, C. Lin, A. Campbell, A. Moulin, and A. A. Herring

EXCESS DEATHS FROM COVID-19

879 Political Determinants of Health: Has COVID-19 Exposed the Worst of It?
G. Chowell and N. Islam

RESEARCH & ANALYSIS

EXCESS DEATHS FROM COVID-19

882 Excess Death Rates by State During the COVID-19 Pandemic: United States, 2020–2023
S. H. Woolf, J. H. Lee, D. A. Chapman, R. T. Sabo, and E. Zimmerman

PERSPECTIVES FROM THE SOCIAL SCIENCES

892 Psychosocial Syndemic Burden, Sexual Behaviors, and Engagement in HIV Prevention Care Among Sexual and Gender Minority Youths: United States, 2022
P. K. Valente, R. Neupane, L. Eaton, and R. J. Watson

HISTORY

903 The History of US Menstrual Health, School Nurses, and the Future of Menstrual Health Equity
S. Bergen, E. D. Maughan, K. E. Johnson, R. Cogan, M. Secor, and M. Sommer

OPEN-THEMED RESEARCH

909 Likelihood of COVID-19 Outbreaks in US Immigration and Customs Enforcement (ICE) Detention Centers, 2020–2021
E. C. Woods, J. R. Andrews, and J. D. Goldhaber-Fiebert

913 Postrelease Risk of Overdose and All-Cause Death Among Persons Released From Jail or Prison: Minnesota, March 2020–December 2021
K. Hill, P. J. Bodurtha, T. N. A. Winkelman, and B. A. Howell

923 Residential Proximity to Oil and Gas Development and Mental Health in a North American Preconception Cohort Study: 2013–2023
M. D. Willis, E. J. Campbell, S. Selbe, M. R. Koenig, J. L. Gradus, Y. I. Nillni, J. A. Casey, N. C. Deziel, E. E. Hatch, A. K. Wesselink, and L. A. Wise

935 Impact of Droughts on Served Drinking Water Disparities in California, 2007–2020
S. Sum

BACKMATTER

OTHER DEPARTMENTS

952 Subscription Form

The Next Generation of LGBTQ+ Health in *AJPH*

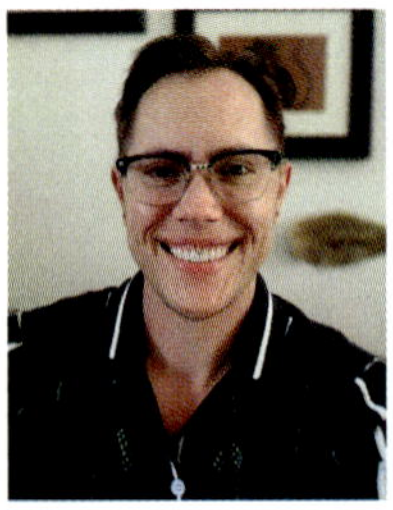
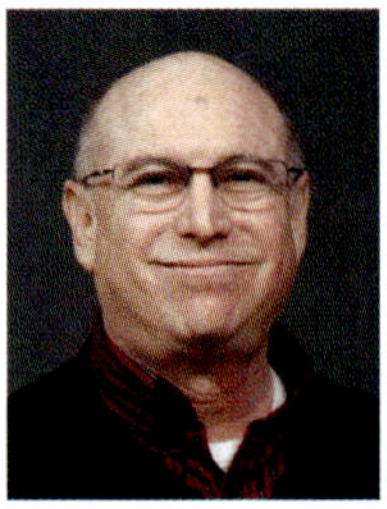

B. Ethan Coston, PhD, MA
AJPH Associate Editor
Stewart Landers, JD, MCP
AJPH Associate Editor Emeritus

AJPH has been a pioneer in the area of LGBTQ+ (lesbian, gay, bisexual, transgender, queer, questioning, asexual, intersex, and other nonheterosexual, noncisgender) people's health as the first mainstream health journal to publish a thematic issue on the topic in June 2001. Since that time, the *Journal* has published hundreds of articles on the subject, building on the growing collection of and access to population-level data, as well as qualitative, community-based, and exploratory analyses and editorials that work to understand the far-reaching impacts of policies, programs, and practices that support or suppress LGBTQ+ health and well-being worldwide.

The *Journal* has recently appointed a new associate editor for LGBTQ+ Health: B. Ethan Coston (they/he). As a transdisciplinary social and behavioral scientist, Coston has more than 15 years' experience in health disparities and equity work. This includes assessing health outcomes and care pathways across gender, sexuality, race/ethnicity, socioeconomic status, disability, neurodivergence, rurality, and age, as well as facing those realities head on through targeted research, education and curriculum development, and health equity and advocacy. Specific areas of Coston's expertise include the causes and health-related consequences of violence, working to promote flourishing mental health and health hardiness for minoritized and systems-affected adolescents and emerging adults, and ongoing work to unearth the historical, sociomedical, and psychiatric construction and regulation of minoritized identities in social, behavioral, and biomedical research.

Coston's appointment comes at a crucial time for LGBTQ+ health in the United States and around the world. In the United States, there has been an alarming increase in anti-LGBTQ+ legislation introduced and passed in the nine years since the Supreme Court's decision on *Obergefell v Hodges* (June 2015).

Although more than one third of 620 bills introduced or carried over in 2024 has focused on limiting or outright banning youth access to gender-affirming health care, nearly all of the laws have far-reaching public health implications and include bills related to educational censorship and exclusion, including allowing misgendering, denying students name and pronoun autonomy, forcibly outing transgender students to their parents, and banning basic gender identity and sexuality and sexual health instruction;

Continued on page e2...

HISTORY CORNER

48 YEARS AGO

Underdevelopment of Health of Working America

[U]sing age-standardized figures, we find far more mortality and morbidity among the working class than among the corporate and upper-middle classes. . . . The main health problems of working America are a result of the lack of power and control over our economic, political, and social institutions by the majority of our population. In that respect, I define social medicine and public health, not only in terms of improving water and sewage systems, or even in terms of improving occupational medicine, but also and primarily (as did the founders of social medicine) in terms of redistributing the economic and political power in our society from the few to the many. Indeed, Virchow, the founder of social medicine, clearly saw the need to merge the medical task with the political and social forces that were mobilized by the emerging working class. Virchow, who joined the first working class revolt of March 18, 1848 in his own city of Berlin, and who also supported the workers' rebellion against the French bourgeoisie in the Paris Commune, clearly saw our task as being political. And in his writings on public health, he concluded that ". . . the very word Public Health shows those who were and still are of the opinion that medicine has nothing to do with politics the magnitude of their error." Moreover, he added that "Medicine is a social science and politics is medicine on a large scale."

From *AJPH*, June 1976, pp. 544–545

sports-related bills that both work to ban transgender athletes from equal participation and attempt to codify sweeping and reductive definitions of sex and gender into law; religious objection laws that allow educators, health care providers, and other public servants to deny LGBTQ+ people care; and legislation to write transgender and intersex people out of state-level definitions (i.e., regarding sex and gender), restrict their ability to update government identification, and ban them from using public, primarily sex-segregated facilities (e.g., public bathrooms).

Unfortunately, these are not only state-level nor Republican-led efforts, although many are. Indeed, the Women's Bill of Rights seeks to erase transgender recognition by the federal government, and the My Child, My Choice Act seeks to prohibit the use of federal education funds unless a teacher requests written parental consent before teaching a lesson specifically related to gender identity, sexual orientation, or transgender studies. National health care bills have also been introduced, including the Protecting Children from Experimentation Act of 2023, which would establish a new federal criminal offense—a fine, a prison term of up to five years, or both—for health care professionals who perform or provide referrals for gender transition procedures on minors.

On a global level, a resurgence of anti-LGBTQ+ legislation is under way in a number of countries. In 2016, the fundamentalist Christian organization Alliance Defending Freedom advised Belize-based groups not to support striking down their colonial-era antisodomy law (https://bit.ly/3xw3hRl), and between 2008 and 2019 they poured more than $38 million into efforts abroad—for example, to oppose same-sex adoption in Austria and the rights of transgender women in France seeking to legally change their gender—by submitting arguments in cases at the European Court of Human Rights (https://bit.ly/3KPgMyB). These efforts have perhaps been most notable in African countries, where US-based anti-LGBTQ+ crusaders (e.g., Christian, Mormon, and Catholic fundamentalists) have found fertile ground for promoting anti-LGBTQ+ hate.

Under Coston's leadership, *AJPH* will be issuing a four-part call for papers series, each on a current topic in LGBTQ+ health that can bring new knowledge and perspectives to how the field of public health addresses the challenges and uses the opportunities of promoting an equitable vision of healthy, thriving LGBTQ+ people and communities. These calls are timed to align with important remembrances, celebrations, and milestones, including a focus on global LGBTQ+ equity for Human Rights Day (December 2024); an exploration of transgender public health for Transgender Day of Visibility (March 2025); a celebration of all things LGBTQ+ joy, well-being, and thriving for LGBTQ+ Pride Month (June 2025); and the first ever special section on intersex people and communities for Intersex Awareness Month (October 2025). The first call for papers can be found at https://ajph.aphapublications.org/callforpapers. AJPH

DOI: https://doi.org/10.2105/AJPH.2024.307751

ORCID iD:
Stewart Landers https://orcid.org/0009-0005-5101-4108

HISTORY CORNER

63 YEARS AGO

Excess Mortality Due to Influenza

Since 1957, the United States has experienced three epidemic waves of Asian influenza. The first two swept the country in the fall of 1957 and the winter of 1958, and led to 60,000 more deaths than would have occurred under normal conditions. The third wave rose abruptly during the first three months of 1960 and produced more than 26,000 excess deaths. These epidemics have been caused by a new antigenic variant of Type A influenza virus, which has been named Type A2. . . . Analysis has shown that the excess deaths from influenza have occurred most markedly among the aged, the chronically ill, and pregnant women. In the most recent epidemic, over three-fourths of the total excess deaths occurred among older persons. Furthermore, the excess deaths were overwhelmingly attributed to two groups: pneumonia-influenza (40 per cent) and cardiovascular-renal disease (46 per cent). Clearly, those who suffer the greatest risk are older persons, particularly those with cardiovascular disorders. For this reason, the U.S. Public Health Service recommends that influenza vaccination for the aged and the chronically ill be made as routine a medical procedure as is immunization of infants against diphtheria or whooping cough.

From *AJPH*, January 1961, p. 107

Advancing, Prioritizing, and Uplifting Equitable Strategies to Improve Black Women's Reproductive Health and Sexuality Wellness

Tiara C. Willie, PhD, MA

ABOUT THE AUTHOR

Tiara C. Willie is with the Department of Mental Health and the Bloomberg American Health Initiative, Johns Hopkins Bloomberg School of Public Health, Baltimore, MD.

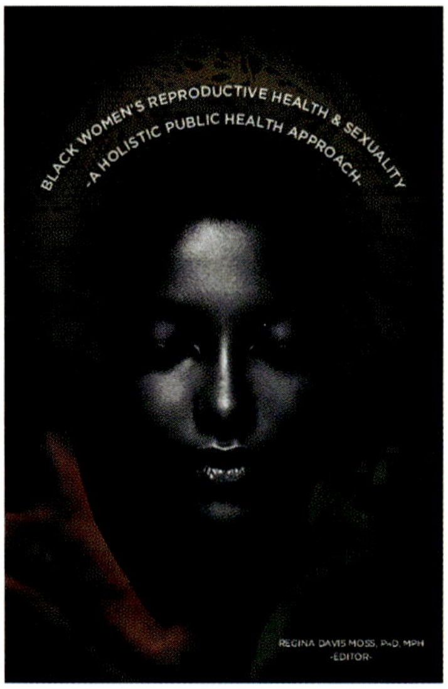

Black Women's Reproductive Health & Sexuality: A Holistic Public Health Approach by Regina Davis Moss, ed.

Washington, DC: American Public Health Association; 2023
Paperback: 444 pp; $64.00
ISBN-10: 087-553340X
ISBN-13: 978-0875533407

"Black women are inherently valuable, that our liberation is a necessity not as an adjunct to somebody else's but because of our need as human persons for autonomy."

—*Combahee River Collective*[1]

For more than 400 years, social–structural determinants have contributed to the dehumanization and deprioritization of Black women's sexual and reproductive health. Rooted in Black feminist theory, intersectionality, a critical theoretical framework, posits that interlocking systems of oppression (e.g., racism, sexism, classism) produce unequal power and privilege for individuals situated at multiple axes of identity,[1–3] and this is especially true for Black women. Racialized, gendered stereotypes about Black womanhood have been perpetuated and weaponized to legitimize their experiences of mistreatment in the health care, housing, and justice systems; the economic exploitation of their reproduction; and the erasure of their victimization in the context of structural and interpersonal violence.

Regina Davis Moss's *Black Women's Reproductive Health & Sexuality: A Holistic Public Health Approach* is a scientifically eloquent love letter to Black women and audiences interested in understanding not only the intersectional social–structural factors contributing to the adverse sexual and reproductive health outcomes among Black women but also the multidisciplinary, multisectoral, and holistic solutions needed for transformative and catalytic change. In four sections comprising 31 chapters, Davis Moss assembled academic and community leaders to author chapters that use quantitative and qualitative intersectionality to develop, implement, and evaluate holistic approaches to Black women's reproductive health and sexuality. These 84 authors are health providers, researchers, advocates, funders and policymakers, and public health practitioners deeply engaged in improving the sexual, maternal, and reproductive health of Black women and girls.

CONTEXTUALIZING HISTORICAL UNDERPINNINGS

The first section of her book is titled "Reborn Not Reformed: Reimagining Research on Black Women's Reproductive Health and Sexuality." This section's collection of chapters is a historical account of how Black women's reproductive health and sexuality have been pathologized from slavery to the post–civil rights era. Recognizing that history is ever present, Davis Moss acknowledges the experimentation on and exploitation of Black women's reproduction during slavery, the suppression of their reproduction during the Jim Crow era through eugenics, the institutionalization of racism in medicine during the civil rights era, and the influx of state-sanctioned compulsory sterilizations and hysterectomies during the post–civil rights era.

Consequently, society's deep-seated adherence to stereotypes about and misrepresentations of Black womanhood has created a context in which Black women's experiences of structural and interpersonal violence are systematically doubted and are not centered in political conversations on sexual and reproductive health. Furthermore, acute and chronic exposure to systems of oppression (e.g., racism, sexism) produces a weathering effect (i.e., "wear and tear" on the body) that can have deleterious and harmful impacts on Black women's maternal and reproductive health. Yet, the section authors' discussion of multilevel holistic recommendations for research, policy, and practice that center Black women and build strategic partnerships with community-based organizations is an uplifting promise of meaningful change.

FILTERING MEDIA PORTRAYALS

Historically, the mass media has directly and indirectly contributed to the devaluation of Black womanhood by perpetuating racialized and gendered myths, narratives, and stereotypes about Black women. In the second section of her book, "Re-embodiment of the Self: Dispelling Myths in Media and Society," Davis Moss and section authors recount how representations and controlling images—such as the Jezebel, the Mammy, the Tragic Mulatto, the Sapphire, the Matriarch, the Welfare Mother, and the Strong Black Woman—have dictated sexual scripts (i.e., guidelines for appropriate sexual behaviors)[4] for Black women. In response to these stereotypes, Black women have engaged in survival strategies, such as subscribing to respectability politics and developing a culture of silence to gain esteem from White America and, in turn, have sacrificed their sexuality and emotions. Recognizing the interconnections between systems of oppression and the mass media, the authors discuss opportunities to combat the sexual oppression of Black women through digital erotic resistance, empowering sexual narratives, and reframing health care education campaigns and television output through a sex-positive lens.

PURSUING ACTIVISM, JUSTICE, AND HEALING

One of the most uplifting sections of Davis Moss's book is the third section, with its strong focus on Black women–led activism in the context of reproductive justice that actively and intentionally rejects reproductive oppression and liberates the experiences of Black birthing people through culturally relevant, person-centered, holistic care. In this section, "Revolutionizing Justice, Activism, and Policy: Creating Movements of True Liberation," Davis Moss and the section authors argue for new and innovative justice frameworks to lead the development of macro- and microlevel interventions to improve the health and well-being of Black women. Specifically, these section authors argue that, given the historical legacy of the sexual and reproductive oppression of Black women, interventions that use justice-oriented reproductive frameworks and liberation health frameworks are critically needed to ensure that transformative change occurs not only at the individual level among Black women but also at the social level in communities, systems, and institutions. Comprehensive legislation and sociopolitical action, such as the Black Maternal Health Momnibus Act, the Kira Johnson Act, and the #MeToo movement, are exemplary solutions that move the needle forward to support the reproductive health of Black women.

BLACK WOMEN'S HEALTH IN THE LIFE STAGES

The fourth and final section of Davis Moss's book, "Recentering Health and Well-Being: Setting the Standard for Holistic Solutions," offers detailed descriptions of the inspiring possibilities of holistic sexual and reproductive health care across the life course for Black women at diverse axes of nativity and sexual identity. This section starts off by highlighting chapters discussing the importance of perinatal care and positive birthing experiences for Black women. The authors argue that health inequities in maternal and infant health will not be removed until birthing work becomes decolonized by encouraging infrastructures to support rebuilding a strong perinatal, midwifery, and lactation workforce; investing in community-based doula models of care; and using trauma-responsive care practices.

The strength of this book is its ability to acknowledge and address intersectional invisibilities[5] in Black maternal and reproductive health. For example, section authors indicate that among birthing inequities of Black people, the unique experiences of migrant Black women are often overlooked, particularly how oppressive migration policies affect their access to sexual and reproductive health care in the United States. Furthermore, this section discusses fertility and infertility considerations among Black women and Black members of the lesbian, gay, bisexual, transgender, queer, and questioning (LGBTQ+) community. Specifically, the historical myth of Black women's hyperfertility has thwarted conversations about infertility and resulted in infertility stigma.

Furthermore, family-building considerations in the Black community need to include members of the LGBTQ+ community, whom may need assistance to conceive; however, the health care system is largely designed for heterosexual patients, and health care providers are often ill equipped to address racism, sexism, and homophobia. This section also covers the absence of discussions of perimenopause and menopause experiences in Black women's health and how chronic stress can exacerbate the weathering effects during this critical period. Public health lifestyle programs need to address the stress–menopause cycle for Black women in midlife.

Coming full circle, this section also considers the importance of comprehensive, sex-positive education and research for not only Black women but Black girls as well. Because society has objectified and adultified Black girls, this group experiences sexual health inequities. Culturally affirming sexual wellness education with a liberation mindset will improve sexual and reproductive health outcomes for Black women and girls by emphasizing strengths-based approaches, such as learning radical self-love, participating in women's circles, and practicing personal healing.

A NEW ERA

Davis Moss's book ends with hope—specifically, with a blueprint of best practices to increase the public health workforce of reproductive justice–informed students, scholars, and practitioners. Although the next generation of health equity scholars are studying and learning, she urges that there be more financial and capacity-building investments in Black women–focused and Black women–led organizations that are advancing work in reproductive health. In the famous words of Audre Lorde, "The master's tools will never dismantle the master's house."[6(p112)] Moving toward a holistic approach to Black women's reproductive health and sexuality requires decolonizing methods, centering the experiences of Black women and girls through justice-oriented and liberatory frameworks, and holding educational and funding institutions responsible for investing in Black women health equity work. AJPH

CORRESPONDENCE

Correspondence should be sent to Tiara C. Willie, 615 N Wolfe St, Office E1148, Baltimore, MD 21205 (e-mail: twillie2@jhu.edu). Reprints can be ordered at https://www.ajph.org by clicking the "Reprints" link.

PUBLICATION INFORMATION

Full Citation: Willie TC. Advancing, prioritizing, and uplifting equitable strategies to improve Black women's reproductive health and sexuality wellness. *Am J Public Health*. 2024;114(9):846–848.

Acceptance Date: June 14, 2024.

DOI: https://doi.org/10.2105/AJPH.2024.307762

ORCID iD:

Tiara C. Willie https://orcid.org/0000-0003-2848-7212

ACKNOWLEDGMENTS

T. C. Willie was supported by the National Institute on Minority Health and Health Disparities, National Institutes of Health (grants K01MD015005, L32MD016555, and R01MD019178).

Note. The funding body did not play a role in this work's interpretation or writing.

CONFLICTS OF INTEREST

The author has no conflicts of interest to declare.

REFERENCES

1. Combahee River Collective. The Combahee River Collective statement: a Black feminist statement. 1977. Available at: https://americanstudies.yale.edu/sites/default/files/files/Keyword%20Coalition_Readings.pdf. Accessed June 24, 2024.
2. Crenshaw K. Mapping the margins: intersectionality, identity politics, and violence against women of color. *Stanford Law Rev.* 1991;43(6):1241–1299. https://doi.org/10.2307/1229039
3. Collins PH. *Black Feminist Thought: Knowledge, Consciousness, and the Politics of Empowerment.* New York, NY: Routledge; 2002.
4. French BH. More than Jezebels and freaks: exploring how Black girls navigate sexual coercion and sexual scripts. *J Afr Am Stud.* 2012;17:35–50. https://doi.org/10.1007/s12111-012-9218-1
5. Purdie-Vaughns V, Eibach RP. Intersectional invisibility: the distinctive advantages and disadvantages of multiple subordinate-group identities. *Sex Roles.* 2008;59:377–391. https://doi.org/10.1007/s11199-008-9424-4
6. Lorde A. The master's tools will never dismantle the master's house. In: Lorde A. *Sister Outsider: Essays & Speeches.* Trumansburg, NY: Crossing Press; 1984:110–113.

School Nurses and the Promotion of Inclusive Menstrual Health

Dominique Tobbell, PhD

ABOUT THE AUTHOR

Dominique Tobbell is with the School of Nursing, University of Virginia, Charlottesville.

See also Bergen et al., p. 903.

Since the introduction of the school nurse role in the early 20th century, school nurses have been an important source of and advocate for children's and adolescents' health care.[1–3] School nurses are often the only consistent source of health care for students, particularly among students from underserved communities, and therefore constitute "a hidden health-care system for children."[4(p232)] Despite school nurses' role in the promotion of individual and population health and their history of partnering with teachers, administrators, families, and caregivers in attending to the diversity of students' health needs, there is a dearth of historical scholarship on school nurses.[1–3] The article by Bergen et al. (p. 903) in this issue of *AJPH* makes a timely and needed intervention.

Bergen et al. analyze the role of school nurses in providing menstrual education to US schoolchildren since the early 20th century, assess the limitations of contemporary menstrual education and the implications for public health, and make recommendations for addressing those challenges. The authors argue that school nurses play an important role in improving menstrual health through the provision of menstrual education but have been historically and persistently underused and underresourced, which hampers their efforts to deliver menstrual education.

The reasons for this include a cultural aversion to open discussion about menstruation, the role of menstrual product manufacturers in providing menstrual education, an absence of national standards for providing menstrual education to school-aged children, and the decentralized nature of US education together with the compounding effects of structural racism on the distribution of educational (and, thus, school nursing) resources. They argue that addressing these limitations and supporting school nurses to provide menstrual education, along with menstrual health care through the establishment of an equity-focused national approach to menstrual health, will lead to improved menstrual health and menstrual health equity in the United States.

Changes in the status of, support for, and scope of practice of school nurses has taken place alongside developments in public health, the shifting health needs of schoolchildren, and changes in the political economy of US education.[1] Nevertheless, as Bergen et al. show, throughout their history, school nurses have been involved in menstrual education. When menstrual product companies assumed a prominent role in the provision of menstrual education materials, beginning in the 1920s, school nurses not only were "conduits" between the corporate materials and their student audiences but, by the 1960s, were also involved in the development of those materials, including educational films. In this way, the authors establish nurses (typically ignored or obscured in scholarship on the subject) as important actors in the proliferation and impact of health education films after World War II.[5]

In providing menstruating adolescents with knowledge to understand and manage their menstruation, school nurses helped to demystify and destigmatize menstruation. Women from diverse backgrounds interviewed about their experiences of menstrual management in the 20th century reported a common belief in the benefits of the menstrual education received in schools and other contexts.[6] As the analysis of Bergen et al. make clear, however, menstrual education has been indelibly shaped by social values and cultural assumptions that have influenced the content of menstrual education as well as the degree to which it was taught. For example, school nursing textbooks and commercially produced educational materials from the 1940s and 1950s sought to reinforce "normative heterosexual expectations around marriage, sex, and family life" (p. 904) even as they challenged older gendered assumptions that menstruation made women inherently weak and unfit for education and work.

Bergen et al. raise important questions about why menstrual education continues to be shaped by attitudes and expectations about gender, sex, and reproduction, including assumptions about normative menstruating bodies. Transgender and nonbinary individuals experience barriers to effective reproductive health care, including symptom management for menstruation, and often encounter discrimination from health care providers because they do not conform to normative expectations of femininity.[7,8] Consequently, it is imperative that school nurses be educated to provide menstrual education and health care that includes and is accessible to menstruating people who identify as transgender or nonbinary and that they are supported in doing so by adequate resources and national standards that are mandated and enforced by the federal Department of Education. National mandates are especially urgent given the number of states that have passed or have pending legislation restricting the rights and health care of transgender youths.[9]

To be sure, it is not just the social and cultural framing of menstrual knowledge that school nurses need to be attentive to: it is also the nature of the knowledge itself. The physiological knowledge historically conveyed in textbooks and health classes has constructed normal, healthy menstruation as a static, 28-day cycle and one in which menstrual pain is assumed to be a normative and routine feature. But as Clancy argues, "The reality is they [menstrual cycles] are malleable, responsive, dynamic,"[10(p7)] and contemporary menstrual education needs to reflect this. The menstrual knowledge conveyed in menstrual education should also address the significant health effects that some menstruating people experience, including severe pain and excessive bleeding, while also addressing the often-debilitating chronic conditions such as endometriosis and premenstrual dysphoric disorder that are associated with menstruation.[10]

As Jones argues, because clinicians have constructed pain as a normal and expected feature of menstruation, the severe pain that is a "symptom of endometriosis is often ignored clinically and culturally,"[11(p559)] contributing to significant delays in diagnosis and medical intervention. Contemporary gender norms regarding pain continue the long history of clinicians dismissing, ignoring, misdiagnosing, and mistreating women's lived experiences of pain.[12] By sharing menstrual knowledge that reflects the variability and complexity of menstruation, and the severe symptoms and chronic conditions that are associated with but *not* normative of menstruation, school nurses can validate students' lived experiences of menstruation and empower those who experience pelvic and menstrual health concerns with knowledge and resources with which to advocate for themselves as they seek health care now and in the future.

Roughly half the school population will experience menstruation, and yet there is an absence of national standards regarding menstrual education (and a dearth of state-level standards)—evidence, as Bergen et al. note, of ongoing gender inequities in the US school system. It is striking, for example, that in school districts, protocols might exist for dealing with a nosebleed or stomachache but not for a student getting their first period at school. This marginalization of menstrual education and health reflects and reinforces the pervasive devaluing of the health experiences of women and other menstruating people—a process that is deeply rooted in history and compounded by the intersectional effects of race, class, and disability.[10,12]

Ultimately, Bergen et al. make clear that establishing a national mandate for menstrual education, along with providing the preparation and resources that will enable school nurses to offer inclusive menstrual education and care to the US school population, is critical to addressing these historical inequities, improving menstrual health, and achieving menstrual equity. AJPH

CORRESPONDENCE

Correspondence should be sent to Dominique Tobbell, University of Virginia School of Nursing, 202 Jeanette Lancaster Way, Charlottesville, VA 22903 (e-mail: dtobbell@virginia.edu). Reprints can be ordered at https://www.ajph.org by clicking the "Reprints" link.

PUBLICATION INFORMATION

Full Citation: Tobbell D. School nurses and the promotion of inclusive menstrual health. *Am J Public Health*. 2024;114(9):849–851.

Acceptance Date: June 19, 2024.

DOI: https://doi.org/10.2105/AJPH.2024.307776

ORCID iD:

Dominique Tobbell https://orcid.org/0000-0002-3855-4370

CONFLICTS OF INTEREST

The author has no conflicts of interest to report.

REFERENCES

1. Hawkins JW, Hayes ER, Corliss CP. School nursing in America—1902–1994: a return to public health nursing. *Public Health Nurs.* 1994;11(6):416–425. https://doi.org/10.1111/j.1525-1446.1994.tb00208.x
2. Apple RD. School health is community health: school nursing in the early twentieth century in the USA. *Hist Educ Rev.* 2017;46(2):136–149. https://doi.org/10.1108/HER-01-2016-0001
3. Houlahan B. Origins of school nursing. *J Sch Nurs.* 2018;34(3):203–210. https://doi.org/10.1177/1059840517735874
4. Willgerodt MA, Brock DM, Maughan ED. Public school nursing practice in the United States. *J Sch Nurs.* 2018;34(3):232–244. https://doi.org/10.1177/1059840517752456

5. Bonah C, Cantor D, Laukotter A, eds. *Health Education Films in the Twentieth Century*. Rochester, NY: University of Rochester Press; 2018. https://doi.org/10.1515/9781787441873
6. Freidenfelds L. *The Modern Period: Menstruation in Twentieth-Century America*. Baltimore, MD: Johns Hopkins University Press; 2009. https://doi.org/10.1353/book.3444
7. Shires DA, Jaffee K. Factors associated with health care discrimination among a national sample of female-to-male transgender individuals. *Health Soc Work*. 2015;40(2):134–141. https://doi.org/10.1093/hsw/hlv025
8. Wingo E, Ingraham N, Roberts SCM. Reproductive health care priorities and barriers to effective care for LGBTQ people assigned female at birth: a qualitative study. *Womens Health Issues*. 2018;28(4):350–357. https://doi.org/10.1016/j.whi.2018.03.002
9. Redfield E, Conron KJ, Mallory C. The impact of 2024 anti-transgender legislation on youth. April 2024. Available at: https://williamsinstitute.law.ucla.edu/wp-content/uploads/2024-Anti-Trans-Legislation-Apr-2024.pdf. Accessed June 2, 2024.
10. Clancy K. *Period: The Real Story of Menstruation*. Princeton, NJ: Princeton University Press; 2023. https://doi.org/10.1515/9780691246826
11. Jones CE. The pain of endo existence: toward a feminist disability studies reading of endometriosis. *Hypatia*. 2016;31(3):554–571. https://doi.org/10.1111/hypa.12248
12. Virdi J. Painful realities. Available at: https://wellcomecollection.org/series/XTg5pRAAACUAP5U5. Accessed June 2, 2024.

Know the Difference Between Jail and Prison? Both Are Associated With Risk of Death

Justin Berk, MD, MPH, MBA, and Lauren Brinkley-Rubinstein, PhD

ABOUT THE AUTHORS

Justin Berk is an assistant professor at the Alpert Medical School at Brown University, Providence, RI. He is the director for the Center for Health and Justice Transformation. Lauren Brinkley-Rubinstein is an associate professor in the Department of Population Health Sciences at Duke University, Durham, NC.

See also Hill et al., p. 913.

AJPH September 2024, Vol. 114, No. 9

Incarceration harms health. Individuals released from carceral facilities have high rates of suicide, overdose, psychiatric hospitalization, and death.[1] Yet, some of the most often cited literature on postrelease mortality precedes the COVID-19 pandemic and the introduction of fentanyl in the illicit drug supply, both adding significant risk to the well-being of incarcerated individuals.

Incarceration takes many different forms. Jails, typically operated by local municipalities, are short-term facilities with rapid turnover and short stays. In contrast, prisons are usually state-run, housing individuals with multiyear sentences. The variability of jails and prisons makes comparing health outcomes challenging; a state-run prison in Washington is very different than a jail in New York City. Even within one state, aggregated data are often unavailable as county- and state-run facilities do not share or make available their data.

NEW FINDINGS IN THE POST–COVID-19, FENTANYL ERA

Yet, in this issue of *AJPH*, Hill et al. (p. 913) become the first to fill a major research gap, simultaneously analyzing statewide jail and prison mortality rates in a post–COVID-19, postfentanyl era. Using linked data sets in Minnesota, the authors compared postrelease standardized mortality rates and overdose fatalities for individuals exposed to jail versus prison.

While the rate of mortality in the general population has gone up over time, the results still confirm that individuals returning to the community from carceral facilities face a disturbingly high mortality rate compared with the general population. Using conservative estimates, the findings are stark: people released from jail or prison were 15.5 times and 28.3 times more likely, respectively, to die from an overdose compared with an age- and gender-matched general Minnesota population. Moreover, these Minnesota cohort data update an absolute mortality rate even higher than the seminal work of Binswanger et al.,[2] though lower than previously calculated standardized mortality rates in very different populations at different times (Table 1).

These findings have significant implications. With more than 10 million individuals cycling through jails in the United States each year, the elevated mortality rate highlights the substantial public health impact of incarceration. Whether they stay one day or 365 days, these data suggest they face a 15-times-higher risk of dying upon release compared with those not incarcerated. The data also reveal that prison stays are associated with an even higher risk of death compared with jails.

UNANSWERED RESEARCH QUESTIONS

However, core research questions remain. One, is the mortality rate for prison higher because of longer length of incarceration or because of something unique to prison exposure? Previous literature—in a prison setting—has found a linear dose–response relationship of time served on mortality: each additional year in prison produced a 15.6% increase in the odds of death for parolees, translating to a two-year decline in life expectancy for each year served in prison.[6] Currently, no data identify if jails have a similar dose–response relationship: a two-day jail incarceration may be very different than a 14-day incarceration.

Second, how does the broader criminal legal system affect these health outcomes? Incarceration is just one aspect of the sequential intercept model of the criminal legal system.[7] A natural follow-up study would compare standardized mortality rates not across just jail and prison but also diversion programs, probation, parole, or other community supervision programs. Other factors, such as recidivism and desistance, may also significantly influence health outcomes.

TABLE 1— Comparison of Previous Literature on Mortality Rate and Overdose Fatalities in US Jails and Prisons

Article	Location	Time Period	Jail or Prison	Sample Size	All-Cause Mortality[a] per 100 000 PY (95% CI)	Overdose Fatalities[a] per 100 000 PY (95% CI)	All-Cause Standardized Mortality Rate, OR (95% CI)	Overdose Standardized Mortality Rate, OR (95% CI)
Hill et al., 2024 (p. 913)	Minnesota	2020–2021	Jail	99 065	1505.3	283.3	1.42 (1.33, 1.51)	15.51 (14.93, 17.11)
			Prison		2169.2	517.6	2.05 (1.69, 2.41)	28.34 (19.71, 37.09)
Lim et al., 2023[3]	New York	2011–2017	Jail	15 797	MOUD: 1160 (940, 1420)	MOUD: 490 (350, 660)	. . .	. . .
					No MOUD: 1430 (1170, 1680)	No MOUD: 830 (640, 1040)	. . .	. . .
Ranapurwala et al., 2022[4]	North Carolina	2000–2018	Prison	229 274	. . .	2 wk postrelease: 960 (646, 1274)	. . .	2 wk postrelease: 46.6 (31.4, 61.8)
					. . .	Overall follow-up: 302 (268, 335)	. . .	Overall follow-up: 14.6 (13.0, 16.6)
Binswanger et al., 2013[5]	Washington	1999–2009	Prison	76 208	737 (708, 766)	167 (153, 181)	3.61 (3.48, 3.73)	10.33 (9.61, 11.10)
Binswanger et al., 2007[2]	Washington	1999–2003	Prison	30 237	. . .	2 wk postrelease: 1840 (1213, 2677)	. . .	2 wk postrelease: 129 (98, 168)
					777 (707, 852)	Overall follow-up: 137 (109, 171)	3.5 (3.2, 3.8)	Overall follow-up: 12.2 (10.2, 14.9)

Note. CI = confidence interval; MOUD = medications for opioid use disorder; OR = odds ratio; PY = person-years.
[a]Data from Hill et al., Ranapurwala et al., and Binswanger et al. are standardized to surrounding general population; Lim et al. data are crude rates at 1-y follow-up.

Finally, how should policymakers interpret these poor health outcomes? These data provide an association without causality. The pathway between carceral setting and death is likely multifactorial. Health care service delivery in carceral settings often lacks evidence-based treatment options (including medications for opioid use disorder [MOUD]), and, without mandatory accreditation bodies or oversight infrastructure, there is substantial heterogeneity among facilities.[8] Moreover, incarceration creates collateral consequences that directly impact social determinants of health. When one has a criminal record, housing, food stamps, employment, and other social services can become more difficult to attain. Limited re-entry service coordination resources and insufficient community supports often exacerbate harms of incarceration.

THE INTERSECTION OF INCARCERATION AND DRUG OVERDOSE

One question has a clear answer: what drives these high mortality rates? The number-one cause of death among people leaving jail (35.9%) and prison (33.1%) is drug overdose.

Upon re-entry from prison, people who use drugs often have reduced tolerance, misjudge dosing, face new adulterants in the illicit drug supply (e.g., xylazine, fentanyl), or lack access to effective treatment therapies without established health care access. The authors confirm these issues (and others) apply to individuals leaving shorter-term facilities (i.e., jails), not just prisons.

Individuals released from carceral facilities—whether jail or prison—face high overdose risk. Indeed, one simulation study in Maryland suggested that nearly 50% of fatal opioid overdoses were with individuals exposed to the criminal legal system.[9] To seriously address the overdose crisis, targeted interventions must not overlook this population.

POLICY IMPLICATIONS

A policy agenda emerges from these findings, focusing on access to both medical and social service relevant care, harm-reduction approaches, and decarceration.

The high rates of opioid overdose demonstrate a clear need for initiation of MOUD in all carceral facilities: jails and prisons alike. Initiation of in-jail treatment has been associated with an 80% decrease in mortality.[3] Despite the robust evidence to support this lifesaving, essential medicine (found to be constitutionally mandated in court cases), uptake of MOUD in carceral facilities remains incredibly low.[10]

In addition, re-entry services are needed to help improve the social and structural determinants of health. This includes housing, food access, employment support (including fair-chance hiring practices), legal services, and social connectedness. Medical programs such as the Transitions Clinic Network work to provide these practices to a patient group most in need.

Harm reduction, now a key pillar of the Substance Abuse and Mental Health Services Administration's Overdose Prevention Strategy, offers an opportunity to save lives and "meet people where they are." Needle exchange programs, safe smoking supplies, low-barrier treatment options, naloxone distribution, drug-checking programs, and safer settings to consume drugs can all help mitigate overdose risk, particularly for this patient population. Harm reduction can also provide a framework to address public health harms of incarceration. How can care be more effectively provided in carceral settings to reduce harms of incarceration? In addition to the need for expansion of MOUD in jails and prisons, facilities can offer programs in HIV, hepatitis C, mental health, cancer screening, and other core improvements in the quality of care. In addition, broader policies that extend beyond harm reduction and eliminate the harmful exposure of carceral settings are needed.

DECARCERATION AS PUBLIC HEALTH INTERVENTION

In 2021, the American Public Health Association published a policy statement that explicitly stated their recommendation of "moving toward the abolition of carceral systems and building in their stead just and equitable structures that advance the public's health."[11] Ruth Wilson Gilmore is often quoted as stating, "Abolition is about presence, not absence. It's about building life-affirming institutions."[12] To assuage the health impact of jails and prisons, public health leaders must work toward the creation of resources to support individuals with addiction, mental health diagnoses, unstable housing, poverty, and other social and structural determinants of health rather than relying on carceral facilities to be safety net providers.

Ultimately, Hill et al. provide a starting point for change. While a Washington State prison differs from a New York City jail, this Minnesota analysis has implications for any state. There is a spectrum of harm between jail and prison that warrants further clarification, but the public health message remains clear: incarceration harms health. AJPH

CORRESPONDENCE

Correspondence should be sent to Justin Berk, 1125 N Main St, Providence, RI 02904 (e-mail: justin_berk@brown.edu). Reprints can be ordered at https://ajph.org by clicking the "Reprints" link.

PUBLICATION INFORMATION

Full Citation: Berk J, Brinkley-Rubinstein L. Know the difference between jail and prison? Both are associated with risk of death. *Am J Public Health*. 2024;114(9):852–855.

Acceptance Date: June 24, 2024.

DOI: https://doi.org/10.2105/AJPH.2024.307777

ORCID iD:

Justin Berk https://orcid.org/0000-0002-2865-7464

CONTRIBUTORS

J. Berk was the initial reviewer of the article and led the writing. L. Brinkley-Rubinstein assisted with the conceptualizing the analysis and the writing.

ACKNOWLEDGMENTS

J. Berk and L. Brinkley-Rubinstein report support from the Lifespan/Brown Criminal Justice Research Program on Substance Use and HIV (R25DA037190). J. Berk reports funding from the National Institute on Drug Abuse (K23DA055695).

CONFLICTS OF INTEREST

The authors report no conflicts of interest.

REFERENCES

1. Brinkley-Rubinstein L. Incarceration as a catalyst for worsening health. *Health Justice*. 2013;1(1):3. https://doi.org/10.1186/2194-7899-1-3
2. Binswanger IA, Stern MF, Deyo RA, et al. Release from prison—a high risk of death for former inmates. *N Engl J Med*. 2007;356(2):157–165. https://doi.org/10.1056/NEJMsa064115
3. Lim S, Cherian T, Katyal M, et al. Association between jail-based methadone or buprenorphine treatment for opioid use disorder and overdose mortality after release from New York City jails 2011–17. *Addiction*. 2023;118(3):459–467. https://doi.org/10.1111/add.16071
4. Ranapurwala SI, Figgatt MC, Remch M, et al. Opioid overdose deaths among formerly incarcerated persons and the general population: North Carolina, 2000–2018. *Am J Public Health*. 2022;112(2):300–303. https://doi.org/10.2105/AJPH.2021.306621

5. Binswanger IA, Blatchford PJ, Mueller SR, Stern MF. Mortality after prison release: opioid overdose and other causes of death, risk factors, and time trends from 1999 to 2009. *Ann Intern Med.* 2013;159(9):592–600. https://doi.org/10.7326/0003-4819-159-9-201311050-00005
6. Patterson EJ. The dose–response of time served in prison on mortality: New York State, 1989–2003. *Am J Public Health.* 2013;103(3):523–528. https://doi.org/10.2105/AJPH.2012.301148
7. Substance Abuse and Mental Health Services Administration. The Sequential Intercept Model (SIM). May 29, 2024. Available at: https://www.samhsa.gov/criminal-juvenile-justice/sim-overview. Accessed June 4, 2024.
8. Alsan M, Yang CS, Jolin JR, Tu L, Rich JD. Health care in US correctional facilities—a limited and threatened constitutional right. *N Engl J Med.* 2023;388(9):847–852. https://doi.org/10.1056/NEJMms2211252
9. Saloner B, Chang HY, Krawczyk N, et al. Predictive modeling of opioid overdose using linked statewide medical and criminal justice data. *JAMA Psychiatry.* 2020;77(11):1155–1162. https://doi.org/10.1001/jamapsychiatry.2020.1689
10. Berk J, Rich J. The Jail and Prison Opioid Project (JPOP). 2021. Available at: https://prisonopioidproject.org. Accessed August 27, 2023.
11. American Public Health Association. Advancing public health interventions to address the harms of the carceral system. American Public Health Association. October 26, 2021. Available at: https://www.apha.org/Policies-and-Advocacy/Public-Health-Policy-Statements/Policy-Database/2022/01/07/Advancing-Public-Health-Interventions-to-Address-the-Harms-of-the-Carceral-System. Accessed July 1, 2024.
12. The End Police Violence Collective. Abolition is public health. January 21, 2022. Available at https://inquest.org/abolition-is-public-health/. Accessed July 1, 2024.

Mass Incarceration and Health Inequities: A Public Health of Consequence, September 2024

Farzana Kapadia, PhD, MPH

ABOUT THE AUTHOR

Farzana Kapadia is the deputy editor of AJPH *and a professor in the Department of Epidemiology, New York University School of Global Public Health, New York.*

See also Berk and Brinkley-Rubinstein, p. 852 and Hill et al. p. 913.

Driven by racist and discriminatory political and ideological motivations focused on punishment rather than prevention or rehabilitation, rates of mass incarceration in the United States are among the highest in the world. The burden of mass incarceration is disproportionately experienced by communities of color and communities made socially and economically vulnerable. The consequences of mass incarceration have profoundly and negatively shaped the health and well-being of incarcerated and formerly incarcerated people as well as their families and communities and society. Recognizing the landscape of structurally racist policies and practices that fuel mass incarceration as well as the social, economic, and health-related inequities that persist after incarceration provides further evidence for the need to disrupt the harms inflicted by mass incarceration.

MASS INCARCERATION IN THE UNITED STATES

The roots of mass incarceration in the United States are intertwined with social, economic, and political upheavals throughout US history. Although these upheavals are disproportionately borne by communities that are marginalized, it is these same communities that bear the disproportionate burden of punitive action and imprisonment. In their report *American History, Race and Prison*, the Vera Institute documents how this cycle continues to play out in the United States—from its settlement, through the post–Civil War period, to the beginning of the mass incarceration era of the 1970s (https://bit.ly/3VzTDFA).

With the expansion of public and then private prisons starting in the 1970s, the overall US incarceration rate grew by more than seven times through 2009 and disproportionately affected people of color, immigrants, and people living in poverty (https://bit.ly/3xxJ4uD). Starting in 2009, criminal justice reform movements to reduce mass incarceration provided modest reductions—0.3% between 2009 and 2010—to the US prison population.[1] Between 2020 and 2022, the COVID-19 pandemic and its social, economic, and political fallout had opposite effects on incarceration rates.[2,3] Specifically, efforts to reduce overcrowding and COVID-19 outbreaks led to reduced prison admissions and expedited release of those imprisoned, resulting in a 14% decrease in the US prison population.[2] However, growing concern about increases in serious crime as well as the persistence of the opioid overdose crisis have led to recent increases in incarceration.[3] As noted by the Sentencing Project, this upward trend in incarceration threatens to reverse efforts to reform and reduce mass incarceration in the United States (https://bit.ly/4bigZVM).

INCARCERATION AND HEALTH INEQUITIES

In January 2020, an *AJPH* supplement (https://bit.ly/4c8CABr) provided far-reaching evidence on how mass incarceration serves as a fundamental driver of health inequities in communities of color and among those made socially and economically vulnerable. Incarceration simultaneously causes and exacerbates poor mental and physical health for those facing incarceration as well as community members residing in neighborhoods with high incarceration rates.[4,5] People who are incarcerated are significantly more likely to already face serious substance use and mental health issues and, although mental and physical care for incarcerated persons is available, the quality and ability to access this care is woefully inadequate.

Despite a constitutional mandate to not inflict "cruel and unusual punishments," incarcerated persons face conditions—physical and sexual violence, inadequate nutrition, unhygienic living conditions, and solitary confinement—that violate basic human rights. Responding to the lack of basic mental and medical health care available to incarcerated persons in California, the US Supreme Court ruled in *Brown v Plata* (563 US 493, 2011) that overcrowding in California prisons placed substantial strain on those prisons. Therefore, to provide adequate access to medical and mental health facilities, the court upheld a ruling to decrease the California prison population by an estimated 46 000 individuals.[6] Although these measures provided a modicum of relief, as noted by Cloud et al., the reality is that "correctional health providers are detached from services, standards, technologies, and ethics of mainstream health systems."[4(p390)]

POSTRELEASE HEALTH INEQUITIES

In 2005, Freudenberg et al. documented the experiences of two groups of vulnerable incarcerated persons—adult women and adolescent males—during their first-year after release from New York City jails.[7] Their findings noted that a greater burden of negative preincarceration life circumstances were prevalent for both groups: poverty, homelessness, previous criminal justice system involvement, poor educational attainment, unemployment, substance use, mental health burdens, violence, and, for women, domestic violence. Layered on top of these circumstances, strained familial and social bonds coupled with lack of housing, employment, health care, and other social supports negatively affected postrelease experiences. In short, inequities before incarceration fueled health inequities after release, increasing the likelihood for recidivism as well as poor health outcomes.

Fast forward 20 years, and the health inequities among people after release from prison and jail have not decreased. In this issue of *AJPH*, Hill et al. (p. 913) present findings based on linked prison, jail, and death records that provide postrelease all-cause and overdose-specific mortality among people leaving jail or prison. Their findings show that rates of overdose deaths among persons released from jail and prison were substantially higher than those of the general Minnesota population. In their editorial, Berk and Brinkley-Rubinstein (p. 852) simultaneously offer potential mechanisms for the drivers of increased all-cause and overdose-specific mortality (i.e., reduced tolerance because of longer prison sentences) and policy and practice recommendations (i.e., expansion of medication for opioid use disorder).

DISRUPTING THE CYCLE

Although the financial costs of mass incarceration are borne by local, state, and federal agencies, the social, economic, and emotional costs are borne by the families, children, and communities of those incarcerated. To break this cycle, preventive efforts at every step of the continuum are required.

First, as a society we need to have honest conversations about what drives crime, how we think about people that engage in criminal activities, and our responses to their acts. Recognizing that structural disadvantages with respect to education, employment, housing, and health are deeply embedded in our society and are the foundational drivers of crime warrants population-level reforms in these areas.

Second, criminal justice reforms across the United States have sought to end a range of structurally racist practices that fuel incarceration rates, including, but not limited to, racial profiling, cash bail, sentencing reform, and overcriminalization (https://bit.ly/4caShls).

Third, redirecting funding to enhance public health and social services to support recently released persons can have significant individual- and population-level benefits. With the passage of the Affordable Care Act (Pub L No. 111-148, 124 Stat. 119, 2010), states are increasingly seeking to enroll incarcerated people in Medicaid before leaving prison and in some instances connect them to case managers and health care providers to prevent gaps in care coverage (https://bit.ly/3VVyRBJ). Ensuring continuity of care is necessary to prevent relapse into substance use and abuse.

Finally, more funding for and development of community-based strategies that can provide a network of community-specific support to prevent recidivism are required. One such strategy is the Maine Prisoner Re-Entry Network (https://re-entrymaine.org/programs), which provides a release plan, housing support, support groups for families of those incarcerated, and mentors to support reentry transitions.

Ending investment in mass incarceration does not threaten community safety. On the contrary, reprioritizing investments in education, economic opportunity, housing, and health care will provide the greatest returns and promote a public health of consequence. AJPH

CORRESPONDENCE

Correspondence should be sent to Farzana Kapadia, PhD, MPH, New York University, School of Global Public Health, 708 Broadway, Room 729, New York, NY 10003 (e-mail: farzana.kapadia@nyu.edu). Reprints can be ordered at https://www.ajph.org by clicking the "Reprints" link.

PUBLICATION INFORMATION

Full Citation: Kapadia F. Mass incarceration and health inequities: a public health of consequence, September 2024. *Am J Public Health*. 2024;114(9):856–858.

Acceptance Date: June 24, 2024.

DOI: https://doi.org/10.2105/AJPH.2024.307780

ORCID iD:

Farzana Kapadia https://orcid.org/0000-0003-3459-767X

CONFLICTS OF INTEREST

The author has no conflicts of interest to disclose.

REFERENCES

1. Guervino P, Harrison PM, Sabol WJ. Prisoners in 2010. 2011. Available at: https://bjs.ojp.gov/content/pub/pdf/p10.pdf. Accessed June 25, 2024.
2. Carson EA. Prisoners in 2020—statistical tables. 2021. Available at: https://bjs.ojp.gov/library/publications/prisoners-2021-statistical-tables. Accessed June 25, 2024.
3. Carson EA, Kluckow R. Prisoners in 2022—statistical tables. 2023. Available at: https://bjs.ojp.gov/library/publications/prisoners-2022-statistical-tables. Accessed June 25, 2024.
4. Cloud DH, Parsons J, Delany-Brumsey A. Addressing mass incarceration: a clarion call for public health. *Am J Public Health*. 2014;104(3):389–391. https://doi.org/10.2105/AJPH.2013.301741
5. Hatzenbuehler ML, Keyes K, Hamilton A, Uddin M, Galea S. The collateral damage of mass incarceration: risk of psychiatric morbidity among nonincarcerated residents of high-incarceration neighborhoods. *Am J Public Health*. 2015;105(1):138–143. https://doi.org/10.2105/AJPH.2014.302184
6. *Brown v Plata*, 563 US 493 (2011).
7. Freudenberg N, Daniels J, Crum M, Perkins T, Richie BE. Coming home from jail: the social and health consequences of community reentry for women, male adolescents, and their families and communities. *Am J Public Health*. 2008;98(9 suppl):S191–S202. https://doi.org/10.2105/ajph.98.supplement_1.s191

Optimizing Wastewater Surveillance: The Necessity of Standardized Reporting and Proficiency for Public Health

Ishi Keenum, PhD, Nancy J. Lin, PhD, Alshae' Logan-Jackson, PhD, Adam J. Gushgari, PhD, Nishita D'Souza, PhD, Joshua A. Steele, PhD, Devrim Kaya, PhD, and Lydia R. Gushgari, PhD

ABOUT THE AUTHORS

Ishi Keenum is with the Civil, Environmental, and Geospatial Department, Michigan Technological University, Houghton. Nancy J. Lin and Alshae' Logan-Jackson are with the Biosystems and Biomaterials Division, National Institute of Standards and Technology, Gaithersburg, MD. Adam J. Gushgari is with Eurofins Pandemic Prevention Services, Sacramento, CA. Nishita D'Souza is with Department of Fisheries and Wildlife, Michigan State University, East Lansing. Joshua A. Steele is with the Department of Microbiology, Southern California Coastal Water Research Project, Costa Mesa, CA. Devrim Kaya is with the School of Public Health, San Diego State University, CA. Lydia R. Gushgari is with SPOC Proteomics, Inc., Scottsdale, AZ.

Wastewater-based surveillance (WBS) has emerged as a valuable tool for public health, allowing a greater understanding of disease prevalence in communities. With historical significance in monitoring polio transmission,[1] WBS gained further prominence in 2020 by enhancing the population-level monitoring of severe acute respiratory syndrome coronavirus 2 (SARS-CoV-2) trends.[2,3] Since then, WBS has been used to track diseases such as influenza,[4] respiratory syncytial virus,[5] norovirus,[6] and mpox. The global implementation of WBS signifies its movement from a research initiative to a staple public health tool, which is especially critical for virus monitoring. However, the diverse methodologies adopted for WBS present challenges. Although each method may address specific stakeholder needs, the lack of standardized reporting guidelines and external validation limits the scope and utility of the data.

A key advantage of WBS is that it enables public health authorities at the state and federal levels to determine where to allocate resources, ideally before a wider spread outbreak. Data aggregation is possible only when metrics such as target concentration and recovery are reported in the same concentrations and with similar driving calculations. This concern is amplified when data from a variety of methods are aggregated at a state, national, or global scale. Therefore, our objective is to promote standardized reporting guidelines in WBS as a critical part of a public health framework.

PROVIDING REAL-TIME ACTIONABLE DATA

WBS provides real-time data on targets (chemical or microbial) to support clinicians, public health response, and the public in general. It can provide an early warning for diseases, as individuals can begin shedding pathogens such as viral particles and microbial cells when they are asymptomatic or presymptomatic.[7,8] It can also provide insight into the presence and transmission of an infection. Historically, WBS has most prominently been implemented for monitoring polio transmission.[1] WBS for SARS-CoV-2 monitoring during the COVID-19 pandemic provided a similar complementary framework for monitoring community disease prevalence when clinical testing was not yet widely available.[2]

Genomic sequencing of target pathogens in wastewater has also proven useful for tracking emerging viral variants of concern and for providing clinicians and public health organizations with information on variants circulating in their community.[9] Furthermore, WBS has improved the ability to develop seasonal viral models for a community. Seasonal models based on clinical data are already established for influenza, but these models do not exist for other viral targets, including respiratory syncytial virus, norovirus, and hepatitis A virus, which is a critical gap in understanding that WBS can fulfill.

WBS enables a dynamic response to a disease outbreak and can be easily pivoted for new and emerging diseases faster than the production of clinical tests. WBS enables public health authorities to have real-time, preclinical data to enable preventive responses in potentially at-risk communities. It can also be used to make sure emergency response personnel have all the necessary personal protective equipment and response tools if called. Thus, WBS fills a previously existing gap in the arsenal of disease-monitoring capabilities.

UNIQUE POPULATION-LEVEL DATA

WBS is fundamentally different from traditional public health testing methods. WBS data can be quantitative, rather than binary, enabling the measurement of the abundance of the pathogen or compound in wastewater. These data allow the direct measurement of a target gene or genes rather than needing to rely on clinical presentation of a disease. WBS captures an integrated sample from the sewered population that can indicate overall disease presence and abundance in a community. It may be particularly useful when traditional public health monitoring is not sensitive enough or there is insufficient infrastructure or funding for traditional public health testing. However, each disease will need to be evaluated for its suitability for WBS monitoring because of variance in shedding rates, persistence in the sewer network, and specificity of the target (primer and probe design). Because of all of these qualities, WBS is a good fit for early detection of outbreaks, tracking the tail end of an outbreak, or seasonal increases and decreases in pathogens in a population. WBS is an important tool to complement, not replace, traditional public health monitoring.

BENEFITS OF PROFICIENCY TESTING

Quality data on disease incidence in a community improve public health monitoring because of increased actionability and confidence. There is potential to adopt similar external quality assessment procedures from the well-established clinical laboratory framework. Accreditation of clinical proficiency testing programs involves a blind analysis on a standardized sample set that is processed identically to real-world samples. Upon submission of the results, the laboratory receives a report that includes the laboratory's results compared with the anticipated values from the reference standard, as well as any necessary corrective actions the laboratory must undertake. Laboratories are routinely reassessed at predefined intervals via externally validated proficiency testing to promote sustained accuracy.

In the United States, the Clinical Laboratory Improvement Amendments maintain and enforce a minimum standard for accuracy, reliability, and quality of laboratory testing focused on the diagnosis, treatment, and prevention of disease. This standard is achieved primarily through workflow-specific evaluations of proficiency and accuracy with a known ground truth as a point of comparison. Efforts in WBS are challenged in this regard because it is difficult to know the absolute concentration of the target, making a ground truth impossible. Laboratory accreditation frameworks exist, including the International Organization for Standardization 17025 framework, which dictates general requirements for testing competency and calibration; however, these are not widely required for public health laboratories. International Organization for Standardization 17025 is a great starting point for all laboratory accreditation, but it will not replace WBS-specific proficiency testing.

The National Institute for Standards and Technology Standards for Wastewater Surveillance Working Group has been developing physical and documentary standards to aid in wastewater surveillance (e.g., development of a DNA standard for mpox assay validation, evaluation of synthetic wastewater for ground truth molecular applications).[10] Current efforts for proficiency testing in WBS have been led by the Ontario Clean Water Agency, which conducts comparative interlaboratory testing on a common sample.[11] Furthermore, the European Union has set a precedent for WBS accreditation with the establishment of the Sewage Core Analysis Group Europe in 2010.[12] This international collaboration gathers multilaboratory WBS data from more than 100 European cities and towns, offering a publicly accessible repository of WBS information as a public health service and resource.

To participate in the Sewage Core Analysis Group Europe program, a laboratory or program must successfully undergo a blind proficiency test, akin to the assessments employed by US clinical laboratory service providers. Using these established resources and expertise could expedite the development of a similar system in the United States. Box 1 synthesizes elements from existing Clinical Laboratory Improvement Amendments and Environmental Protection Agency drinking water microbiology analysis as elements that are critical for reporting.

Currently, WBS laboratory processes operate without a federally mandated regulatory framework. Although the National Wastewater Surveillance System (NWSS) currently serves as the primary data repository for WBS data in the United States, it relies on self-reported data that practitioners

BOX 1— Existing Clinical and Environmental Proficiency and Reporting Standards and Their Identified Relevance to Wastewater-Based Surveillance (WBS)

Sample Processing Stage	Relevant CLIA Recording Requirements[13]	Relevant EPA Laboratory Certification for Microbiology in Drinking Water[14]	WBS Applicable Parameters
Preanalytic sampling and transport	Sample location, time, date, sample storage and preservation, conditions for transportation	Site location, sample type, name of sampler, date and time, chain of custody	Sample location, time, date, sample storage and preservation, conditions for transportation
During sample processing	• Control procedures and corrective action to take when calibration or controls fail, reportable range for test results in the test system as established • Reference or typical intervals • Established system for where to enter results for a specific test or step in the workflow	• Date and time of analysis • Inclusion and analysis of controls, including positives and negatives • Method conducted • Laboratory and signature of person performing analysis	• Date and time of analysis • Inclusion and handling of positive and negative controls • Method conducted • Laboratory and signature of person performing analysis
Reporting	• Results reported from collected data • Test report date and assays run • Pertinent "normal" values	• Maintain records for 5 y, including raw data calculations and quality control data	• Results reported from collected data • Report raw data, calculations, and quality control data

Note. CLIA = Clinical Laboratory Improvement Amendments; EPA = Environmental Protection Agency.

generate without external validation. In the process of developing these programs, it is crucial to strike a balance between establishing a regulatory framework to uphold data quality and ensuring that the demands on WBS laboratories are not unduly onerous.

The expenses associated with laboratory accreditation processes ultimately contribute to the per sample cost for end users. This expense raises the concern of potentially offsetting the cost-effectiveness that is currently a fundamental advantage of the WBS process. The establishment of an external standardized evaluation framework and proficiency testing is an essential step in the evolution of the field, particularly as WBS continues to gain traction and expand its future analytical capability.

REPORTING GUIDELINES

Developing data that are comparable across districts and time points is critical for building a robust monitoring network and enables individual laboratories to track performance as they improve or expand their targets of interest. Comparable data also allow data aggregation and reuse as well as a well-informed regional public health response. Most recommendation guidelines have focused primarily on the comparability of generated data and not on the actionability that additional data collection can provide. Both of these are key elements that are needed to maximize the utility of WBS.

Guidelines exist for environmental monitoring via digital PCR (polymerase chain reaction) and qPCR (quantitative PCR); however, these guidelines do not focus on a public health–based framework[15,16] These stakeholder-developed guidelines have promoted workflow transparency in environmental monitoring while facilitating method innovation. However, researchers have repeatedly identified the need for these practices to be enforced by journals as well as data repositories to ensure they are followed. Although these guidelines are not focused on a public health–based framework, best practices and lessons learned from them could serve to inform the development of WBS reporting guidelines, as was suggested by McClary et al.[17] This framework can be modified to remain target neutral while also incorporating elements of environmental sampling known to affect reported concentrations.

Reporting for WBS in the United States is heavily driven by programs such as NWSS. In addition to reporting what NWSS requires, which includes laboratory processing steps, including concentration method, nucleic acid extraction method, and recovery, laboratories should include any additional data or metadata critical for public health authorities to generate actionable insights. Common, open reporting guidelines would serve to clarify and standardize what (e.g., units) should be reported and how (e.g., concentrations). WBS implementers must strike a balance between speed, data quality assurance and quality control, and actionability. Reporting guidelines that cover the entire WBS workflow must be easily accessible to laboratories and, ideally, should be streamlined across organizations within a country and across countries for global surveillance efforts.

Global efforts such as the public health environmental surveillance open data model can aid in generating interoperable data-handling pipelines across sites.[18] Furthermore, reporting will improve WBS quality if the model can provide more information about the collected sample, including metadata (e.g., weather conditions, which can affect sewage dilution rate) and the exact sample collection point for sewershed mapping.

CHALLENGES TO STANDARDIZATION

Every sewer system is unique because of factors such as its size, demographics served, location, age, and sewer contributors, making standardizing WBS a daunting task. Moreover, WBS programs and monitoring laboratories have constraints that affect monitoring frequency, number of sampling points, and methodologies. This is further compounded by challenges such as supply chain shortages that can lead to using method substitutes. The inherent variety present in WBS systems and data generation further emphasizes the critical role that proficiency testing programs could play in WBS. Many methods can generate valid WBS results[19]; therefore, verifying that a laboratory is applying its selected method of choice accurately can greatly help to improve the robustness and utility of generated data.

Method-specific guidance must also be developed to guide new WBS implementers away from common pitfalls. The National Institute of Standards and Technology and Technology Standards for Wastewater Surveillance Working Group is working to develop high-level guidelines for the most common WBS methodologies to aid in this effort. This, in conjunction with common reporting guidelines, will aid in pushing WBS to new discoveries. Providing best practices for data and metadata reporting will facilitate comparable, reusable data and lay the foundation for future methodological standards when the field is ready for them.

THE FUTURE IS BRIGHT

We are just beginning to realize the extensive public health benefits of WBS, particularly in terms of tracking disease prevalence and guiding targeted public health interventions. In addition, WBS is being expanded to monitor the prevalence of antimicrobial resistance genes in wastewater to support the global fight against antibiotic and antimicrobial resistance. Although we have focused here on microbial targets, WBS has been applied to chemical targets for applications such as illicit drugs, indicators of vaccinations for rate measurement, antiretrovirals, and medicines used for home management of disease. An integration of microbial and chemical WBS will enable the expanded application of WBS in public health and will usher in a more advanced understanding of targets, such as pathogens (e.g., SARS-CoV-2, Coxsackievirus) and antiretroviral medications (e.g., Paxlovid, efavirenz). Reporting guidelines and proficiency testing could be expanded to encompass chemical targets in addition to microbial targets to facilitate the integration of multiple data types to address complex public health issues.

The types of laboratories performing WBS have expanded since the start of the COVID-19 pandemic, enhancing the capability of WBS. Initially, the testing laboratories reporting to NWSS included primarily academic, environmental, and private sector organizations. As the pandemic progressed, public health laboratories and health departments developed the capability to operate in the WBS space. Such laboratories are now equipped to monitor wastewater for targets as well as to analyze and interpret data. This expansion of participants in NWSS and WBS in general highlights the importance of the requirements for data reporting and data validation to be streamlined across organizations, easily accessible, and nonlaborious to be adopted throughout the field. The development of standards for WBS requires a community-driven effort with input from all key stakeholders. We have focused on reporting guidelines here, but standards are needed to support the full WBS workflow. Different types of standards, such as consensus-based documentary standards and reference materials, can be used in concert to support WBS.

CONCLUSIONS

WBS is a valuable public health tool that can be strengthened by the integration of external validation frameworks and reporting guidelines. It provides novel data that can inform the public health response. The diversity of individuals and organizations participating in WBS strengthens the field, as it introduces new viewpoints and utility for monitoring targets. AJPH

CORRESPONDENCE

Correspondence should be sent to Ishi Keenum, PhD, Civil, Environmental, and Geospatial Department, Michigan Technological University, 1400 Townsend Dr, Dow 870, Houghton, MI 49931 (e-mail: imkeenum@mtu.edu). Reprints can be ordered at https://www.ajph.org by clicking the "Reprints" link.

PUBLICATION INFORMATION

Full Citation: Keenum I, Lin NJ, Logan-Jackson A, et al. Optimizing wastewater surveillance: the necessity of standardized reporting and proficiency for public health. *Am J Public Health*. 2024;114(9): 859–863.

Acceptance Date: June 10, 2024.

DOI: https://doi.org/10.2105/AJPH.2024.307760

ORCID iD:
Ishi Keenum https://orcid.org/0000-0002-5441-4634

CONTRIBUTORS

I. Keenum conceptualized the editorial and wrote the first draft. N. J. Lin, A. Logan-Jackson, A. J. Gushgari, N. D'Souza, J. A. Steele, and D. Kaya wrote, reviewed, and edited the editorial. L. R. Gushgari contextualized, edited, and reviewed the editorial.

ACKNOWLEDGMENTS

Logan and Lin were supported in part by the Science and Technology Directorate of the US Department of Homeland Security with the National Institute of Standards and Technology (NIST; interagency agreement FTST-22-FT006-000-000).

The authors would like to thank the NIST-led Standards for Wastewater Surveillance Working Group for bringing the authors together and leading the efforts in the development of standards for wastewater-based surveillance.

CONFLICTS OF INTEREST

The authors report no known conflicts of interest.

REFERENCES

1. Más Lago P, Gary HE Jr, Pérez LS, et al. Poliovirus detection in wastewater and stools following an immunization campaign in Havana, Cuba. *Int J Epidemiol*. 2003;32(5):772–777. https://doi.org/10.1093/ije/dyg185
2. Medema G, Heijnen L, Elsinga G, Italiaander R, Brouwer A. Presence of SARS-coronavirus-2 RNA in sewage and correlation with reported COVID-19 prevalence in the early stage of the epidemic in the Netherlands. *Environ Sci Technol Lett*. 2020;7(7):511–516. https://doi.org/10.1021/acs.estlett.0c00357
3. Bivins A, North D, Ahmad A, et al. Wastewater-based epidemiology: global collaborative to maximize contributions in the fight against COVID-19. *Environ Sci Technol*. 2020;54(13):7754–7757. https://doi.org/10.1021/acs.est.0c02388
4. Wolfe MK, Duong D, Bakker KM, et al. Wastewater-based detection of two influenza outbreaks. *Environ Sci Technol Lett*. 2022;9(8):687–692. https://doi.org/10.1021/acs.estlett.2c00350
5. Hughes B, Duong D, White BJ, et al. Respiratory syncytial virus (RSV) RNA in wastewater settled solids reflects RSV clinical positivity rates. *Environ Sci Technol Lett*. 2022;9(2):173–178. https://doi.org/10.1021/acs.estlett.1c00963
6. Boehm AB, Wolfe MK, White BJ, et al. Human norovirus (HuNoV) GII RNA in wastewater solids at 145 United States wastewater treatment plants: comparison to positivity rates of clinical specimens and modeled estimates of HuNoV GII shedders. *J Expo Sci Environ Epidemiol*. [Epub ahead of print August 7, 2023]. https://doi.org/10.1038/s41370-023-00592-4
7. Betancourt WQ, Schmitz BW, Innes GK, et al. COVID-19 containment on a college campus via wastewater-based epidemiology, targeted clinical testing and an intervention. *Sci Total Environ*. 2021;779:146408. https://doi.org/10.1016/j.scitotenv.2021.146408
8. Olesen SW, Imakaev M, Duvallet C. Making waves: defining the lead time of wastewater-based epidemiology for COVID-19. *Water Res*. 2021;202:117433. https://doi.org/10.1016/j.watres.2021.117433
9. Vo V, Tillett RL, Papp K, et al. Use of wastewater surveillance for early detection of Alpha and Epsilon SARS-CoV-2 variants of concern and estimation of overall COVID-19 infection burden. *Sci Total Environ*. 2022;835:155410. https://doi.org/10.1016/j.scitotenv.2022.155410
10. National Institute of Standards and Technology. Wastewater surveillance. Available at: https://www.nist.gov/programs-projects/wastewater-surveillance. Accessed July 2, 2024.
11. Chik AHS, Glier MB, Servos M, et al. Comparison of approaches to quantify SARS-CoV-2 in wastewater using RT-qPCR: results and implications from a collaborative inter-laboratory study in Canada. *J Environ Sci (China)*. 2021;107:218–229. https://doi.org/10.1016/j.jes.2021.01.029
12. European Union Drugs Agency. Wastewater analysis and drugs—a European multi-city study. Available at: https://www.emcdda.europa.eu/publications/html/pods/waste-water-analysis_en. Accessed October 30, 2023.
13. Laboratory Requirements. 42 CFR, part 493 (1990). Available at: https://www.ecfr.gov/current/title-42/part-493. Accessed March 26, 2024.
14. Environmental Protection Agency. *Manual for the Certification of Laboratories Analyzing Drinking Water: Criteria and Procedures Quality Assurance*, Fifth Edition. 2005. Available at: https://nepis.epa.gov/Exe/ZyPDF.cgi?Dockey=30006MXP.txt. Accessed July 2, 2024.
15. Bustin SA, Benes V, Garson JA, et al. The MIQE guidelines: minimum information for publication of quantitative real-time PCR experiments. *Clin Chem*. 2009;55(4):611–622. https://doi.org/10.1373/clinchem.2008.112797
16. Borchardt MA, Boehm AB, Salit M, Spencer SK, Wigginton KR, Noble RT. The environmental microbiology minimum information (EMMI) guidelines: qPCR and dPCR quality and reporting for environmental microbiology. *Environ Sci Technol*. 2021;55(15):10210–10223. https://doi.org/10.1021/acs.est.1c01767
17. McClary-Gutierrez JS, Aanderud ZT, Al-Faliti M, et al. Standardizing data reporting in the research community to enhance the utility of open data for SARS-CoV-2 wastewater surveillance. *Environ Sci (Camb)*. 2021;9:10.1039/d1ew00235j. https://doi.org/10.1039/d1ew00235j
18. PHES-ODM validation documentation. Available at: https://validate-docs.phes-odm.org/index.html. Accessed March 21, 2024.
19. Pecson BM, Darby E, Haas CN, et al. Reproducibility and sensitivity of 36 methods to quantify the SARS-CoV-2 genetic signal in raw wastewater: findings from an interlaboratory methods evaluation in the US. *Environ Sci (Camb)*. 2021;7:504–520. https://doi.org/10.1039/D0EW00946f

Educational Outcomes Are an Underused Metric for Child and Life Course Health

Nadav L. Sprague, MPH, Charles C. Branas, PhD, Andrew G. Rundle, DrPH, and Pam Factor-Litvak, PhD

ABOUT THE AUTHORS

Nadav L. Sprague is a PhD candidate in epidemiology at Columbia University's Mailman School of Public Health, New York, NY. Charles C. Branas, Andrew G. Rundle, and Pam Factor-Litvak are professors in Columbia University's Mailman School of Public Health.

We explore the reciprocal relationship between education and health. By combining the often siloed literature bases on how children's health affects their educational outcomes[1] and how children's educational outcomes shape their life course health,[2] we provide a comprehensive conceptual model for this reciprocal relationship. The potential for using educational data to enhance public health understanding is significant, particularly in high-income countries such as the United States, where the creation of databases of de-identifiable data for all students' educational outcomes is feasible.

Such databases could encompass a wide range of anonymized information, including academic performance metrics (e.g., grades and standardized test scores), attendance, disciplinary incidents (e.g., detention, suspensions, and expulsions), and socioeconomic demographic data. These databases could also be connected to medical records by a third party (to preserve anonymity) and used to create predictive models for an array of health outcomes. Using this comprehensive information offers a more inclusive and insightful approach to public health analysis, encompassing data from every student in a country's educational system rather than relying solely on smaller cohorts that have more detailed biometric data but are often poorly representative compared with these national data's potential.

Despite the wealth of public health information that educational data can offer, educational variables (e.g., grades, attendance, and test results) as indicators for health outcomes often remain sidelined in health studies and are commonly used only in health fields such as educational psychology and school-based health (see the Appendix for further reading, available as a supplement to the online version of this article at https://www.ajph.org). In fact, in a 2011 review conducted by the World Health Organization (WHO), there were only 53 studies that examined the association between health and education indicators in high-income countries.[3] This scarcity in research has persisted over the years, hindering the integration of educational outcomes as proxies for health in research endeavors, despite the wealth of accessible data in educational systems, which include grades, standardized test results, attendance records, and dropout rates. The underuse of these readily available educational data in health research is a missed opportunity and hampers our ability to comprehensively understand and address health disparities and outcomes.

We expand on the 2011 WHO report and explore the current evidence base on the connections between academic success (i.e., achieving desired educational goals and outcomes in an academic setting), educational attainment (i.e., highest level of education an individual has completed), and health outcomes. From there, we develop a conceptual model of the multistage relationship between education and health. Based on that framework, we discuss how educational and health disparities reinforce one another.

Our aim is to address the critical need to reexamine the relationship between education and health and show the importance of considering educational attainment and academic success as valuable proxy variables for health outcomes in the scientific literature. By recognizing and using the profound relationship between educational factors and health outcomes, researchers could more regularly use these educational factors as proxies for health variables because of the potential wealth of data. Through the increased integration of educational data into public health research, we aim to advance strategies to promote preventive medicine and enhance overall well-being, thereby contributing to the holistic improvement of public health initiatives.

ACADEMIC SUCCESS AND HEALTH OUTCOMES

There is a multistage relationship between academic success, educational attainment, and health outcomes. As shown in Figure 1, children's health significantly influences their school attendance and concentration levels, ultimately influencing academic performance and educational attainment.[1,4,5] Therefore, children's health should be considered an upstream determinant of academic success and educational attainment. Yet, a well-established knowledge base documents academic success and educational attainment as upstream determinants of health.[6] Numerous studies conclude that children's academic performance and educational attainment affect their health outcomes throughout their life course (see the Appendix for further reading). As shown in Figure 1, education contributes to both childhood and life course health through the pathways of literacy, health knowledge, and healthy behaviors. Education also shapes life course, as well as intergenerational, health through social, psychological, and employment-related pathways (see the Appendix for further reading). We elaborate on this multistage relationship, discussing how children's health affects their educational outcomes and, in turn, how educational outcomes affect life course health outcomes.

Children's Health Impact on Education

In the first stage of this relationship, children's health status drives school attendance, ultimately influencing academic performance and educational attainment (Figure 1).[1,4,5] A well-established evidence base suggests an association between childhood chronic illness and decreases in school attendance, which may lead to decreases in academic success.[1,5]

This relationship has been well documented since the 1980s.[5] A landmark study in North Carolina of 270 children during the 1981–1982 school year found that students with chronic illnesses had more than double the number of days absent than did their classmates without any chronic illness.[5] In this study, the students suffered with one of the following chronic health conditions: arthritis, blood disorder, acquired or congenital cardiac disease, chronic bowel disease, chronic lung disease, cystic fibrosis, diabetes, epilepsy, hemophilia, sickle cell disease, or spina bifida. The same study found that chronically ill children scored significantly lower on national achievement tests than did their healthy counterparts.[5]

This trend has proven consistent over time, as a study using 2008 data from 2183 North Carolina children found significant associations between children's oral health and their educational outcomes.[4] The study found that children with poor oral health were nearly three times more likely to miss school because of dental pain and nearly 70% more likely to have poor school performance than were their counterparts with good oral health.[4]

Similar findings have been documented throughout the United States, Canada, South America, and Europe (see the Appendix for further reading).[7]

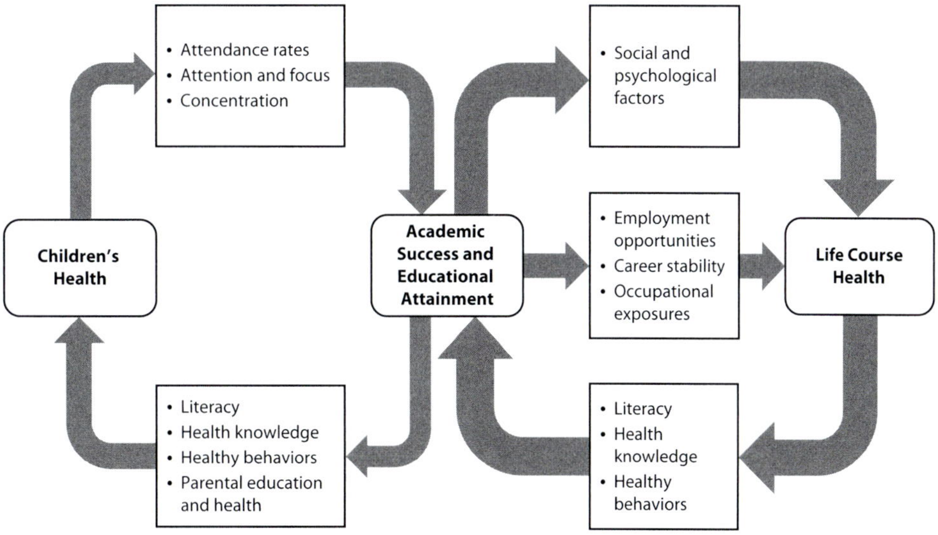

FIGURE 1— Conceptual Model of the Pathways Linking the Multistage Relationship of Health and Education

A study conducted in Argentina found that children's academic performance is influenced by their health status of the previous academic year.[7] Presumably, this phenomenon may occur because students missed core concepts from the previous school year and therefore are further behind classmates. The evidence is clear and consistent that children's health status directly affects educational outcomes. Consequently, children's health should be considered an upstream determinant of educational success.

Education Impact on Life Course Health

In public health, academic success and educational attainment are more commonly discussed as upstream social determinants of health.[6] Educational success has strong and significant effects on health outcomes throughout the life course.[6] We discuss the three interrelated pathways that connect academic success and educational attainment to life course health outcomes (Figure 1).[2]

Increasing literacy, health knowledge, and healthy behaviors. A substantial body of evidence, including numerous systematic reviews, suggests that schooling significantly affects children's literacy, health knowledge, and healthy behaviors.[8,9] Literacy, healthy behaviors, and health knowledge are essential for healthy lives. One systematic review, which assessed 24 peer-reviewed articles on the topic, concluded that children who struggle with literacy have worse health behaviors than do their counterparts with age-standard literacy.[9] Other systematic reviews have documented that children with low health literacy and adults with low general literacy have poorer health outcomes throughout the life course (see the Appendix for further reading). Another systematic review examined 20 peer-reviewed articles and concluded that reduced literacy is a direct barrier to health knowledge, as most medical understanding requires the ability to read (e.g., instructions on pill bottles, e-mail communication with medical providers, and health information pamphlets).[10]

Both studies and reviews documented that classroom and school environments greatly influence children's health behavior (see the Appendix for further reading). Healthy behaviors learned at school include socialization, self-regulation, and physical activity (see the Appendix for further reading).[11] The health behaviors learned in childhood are often associated with long-term health behaviors and health outcomes throughout the life course.[11,12]

Current research suggests that more highly educated individuals (i.e., those who have completed more levels of education) are more likely to have higher rates of positive health behaviors (e.g., physical activity and healthy diet) and lower rates of adverse health behaviors (e.g., cigarette smoking and poor sleeping patterns) than are their counterparts.[11,13,14] Thus, academic success and educational attainment influence life course health outcomes by improving literacy, increasing health knowledge, and promoting healthy behaviors.

Enhancing employment opportunities, financial and occupational stability, and health. Educational outcomes influence health outcomes by shaping employment opportunities.[2] Higher academic success and educational attainment are associated with greater employment opportunities, increased job security, and more control over personal work environment (see the Appendix for further reading). Employment opportunities are directly related to economic resources and economic security, which in the United States are directly correlated to life course health outcomes.[2,15,16] Additionally, more highly educated individuals are more likely to have employment with healthier work environments, better health-related benefits (e.g., health insurance, employee assistance programs, preventive services, and medical savings plans), higher compensation, and lower exposures to occupational hazards.[2,17,18] All these factors also reduce the prevalence and severity of chronic stress more effectively among more highly educated individuals than among their less-educated counterparts.[2]

Chronic stress is an important health metric, as it significantly impairs a wide array of health outcomes (see the Appendix for further reading). This is exemplified by a meta-analysis of 23 cohort studies encompassing 222 120 participants, which revealed a significant association between long working hours and diabetes among the low socioeconomic status group (risk ratio [RR] = 1.29; 95% confidence interval [CI] = 1.06, 1.57), whereas no significant association was observed in the high socioeconomic group (RR = 1.00; 95% CI = 0.80, 1.25).[19] As educational attainment is a facet of socioeconomic status, this study demonstrates how education provides enhanced employment opportunities, which in turn profoundly affect health outcomes. In summary, academic success and educational attainment increase employment opportunities, directly and indirectly bearing on life course health outcomes.

Improving health through social and psychological factors. Lastly, academic success and educational attainment influence life course health outcomes by influencing self-efficacy, social status, and social support.[2,20] The current evidence base suggests that higher-quality education (i.e., educational systems or programs that provide superior learning experiences, resources, and opportunities for students) is associated with higher rates of self-efficacy and feelings of self-control, which in turn improve health behaviors and health outcomes.[2,20,21] Additionally, research has demonstrated that higher levels of academic success and educational attainment are associated with higher levels of socioeconomic status and social support.[2] Higher levels of social support improve both mental and physical health outcomes.[22]

It is reasonable to assume that individuals are in social networks of similarly educated people (e.g., co-workers and grade school or university classmates). Presumably, then, more highly educated individuals are in social networks that are more likely to encourage healthier behaviors and that may be financially capable of supporting network members in need. Therefore, individuals with higher academic success and educational attainment are likely to have better life course health outcomes through increased self-efficacy, social status, and social support.

US EDUCATIONAL DISPARITIES

The United States has significant educational disparities that mirror and reinforce health disparities. The complex multistage relationship between an individual's academic success, educational attainment, and health outcomes reinforces both educational and health disparities cyclically. In the United States, health and educational inequities disproportionately affect low-income, Black, and Hispanic youths compared with their high-income, White, and non-Hispanic counterparts (see the Appendix for further reading). These inequities result from numerous other disparities, such as classroom sizes, classroom and school funding, teacher biases, home environments, school built and food environments, and access to supplementary resources (see the Appendix for further reading). Although nominal reductions in the socioeconomic educational gap have been documented, projections predict this gap will not close until after the year 2150.[23,24] However, these analyses were conducted before the COVID-19 pandemic, which has been documented to exacerbate educational disparities, and did not incorporate climate change, which is also believed to increase such disparities.[25,26]

The same nominal improvements in racial and ethnic disparities have not been documented.[27,28] One study investigated the trends of the non-Hispanic White–Hispanic White and White–Black educational gaps from 1986 to 2014 and found that Black students persistently enroll at increasingly less selective institutions than do their White counterparts.[27] The study also found that the non-Hispanic White–Hispanic White educational gap remained nearly unchanged over the 28 years of the study.[27] Moreover, these studies on socioeconomic, racial, and ethnic disparities did not consider potential threat-multiplying events (e.g., the COVID-19 pandemic and climate change), which may further exacerbate these educational disparities.[29,30] In summary, there are well-established, persistent socioeconomic, racial, and ethnic educational disparities in the United States that reinforce mirroring health disparities.

A CALL FOR MORE EDUCATIONAL DATA

As educational and health disparities mutually reinforce each other and are both expected to be exacerbated by compounding threats such as climate change, there is a critical need to position educational variables as essential proxies in health research and life course health prediction. Several studies in both the medical science and educational fields have documented correlations between race, ethnicity, family income, health outcomes, and educational disparities, underscoring the complex interplay between these factors.[31–33]

Despite the significant potential that educational data hold for enriching public health understanding, their underuse persists. We advocate the prioritization of educational outcomes as integral components of health research because they offer invaluable insights for gauging child health status and predicting life course health trajectories. The absence of comprehensive national, school district, and state-level educational data is hindering progress in both education and health domains. The lack of easily accessible educational data (other than standardized test scores) from governmental sources for researchers is detrimental to both educational and health research, as it negatively affects the outcomes in both crucial domains.

More comprehensive inclusion of educational data in health studies necessitates the establishment of robust mechanisms that facilitate access to national or regional data. Embracing databases of de-identifiable data on students' educational records on broader scales, especially in higher-income countries with the capacity to create them, such as the United States, presents a distinctive opportunity to enhance public health and preventive medicine initiatives. With a thorough integration of educational data into health research, researchers can harness a wealth of information to advance strategies addressing health disparities and fostering improved public health outcomes.

CONCLUSIONS

In light of the evidence we have presented, it is clear that the use of educational data in health research is crucial yet underappreciated. Child health is an upstream determinant of education, and education is a clear upstream determinant of health. This relationship is often intensified, as communities often face both health and educational disparities and crises in a syndemic fashion. However, educational data are often relegated to the periphery in health research and remain an untapped source of valuable insights. Health researchers, policymakers, and practitioners must incorporate educational data more regularly in their work, as health metrics are essential for promoting well-being and preventing disease. AJPH

CORRESPONDENCE

Correspondence should be sent to Nadav L. Sprague, MPH, Department of Epidemiology, Columbia University Mailman School of Public Health, 722 W 168th St, New York, NY 10032 (e-mail: NLS2171@cumc.columbia.edu). Reprints can be ordered at https://www.ajph.org by clicking the "Reprints" link.

PUBLICATION INFORMATION

Full Citation: Sprague NL, Branas CC, Rundle AG, Factor-Litvak P. Educational outcomes are an underused metric for child and life course health. *Am J Public Health*. 2024;114(9):864–869.

Acceptance Date: June 14, 2024.

DOI: https://doi.org/10.2105/AJPH.2024.307761

ORCID iD:

Nadav L. Sprague https://orcid.org/0000-0002-9698-9962

CONTRIBUTORS

N. L. Sprague visualized and wrote the first draft of the editorial. N. L. Sprague, C. C. Branas, and P. Factor-Litvak conceptualized the work. C. C. Branas, A. G. Rundle, and P. Factor-Litvak supervised the work. All authors contributed to writing, reviewing, and editing the editorial.

ACKNOWLEDGMENTS

The authors acknowledge and extend heartfelt gratitude to all teachers and educators whose dedication and passion make a significant difference in the lives of students.

CONFLICTS OF INTEREST

The authors have no conflicts of interest to disclose.

REFERENCES

1. Wolfe BL. The influence of health on school outcomes: a multivariate approach. *Med Care*. 1985; 23(10):1127–1138. https://doi.org/10.1097/00005650-198510000-00001
2. Braveman P, Egerter S, Williams DR. The social determinants of health: coming of age. *Annu Rev Public Health*. 2011;32:381–398. https://doi.org/10.1146/annurev-publhealth-031210-101218
3. Suhrcke M, de Paz Nieves C. The impact of health and health behaviours on educational outcomes in high-income countries: a review of the evidence. 2011. Available at: https://iris.who.int/handle/10665/345467. Accessed June 23, 2024.
4. Jackson SL, Vann WF Jr, Kotch JB, Pahel BT, Lee JY. Impact of poor oral health on children's school attendance and performance. *Am J Public Health*. 2011;101(10):1900–1906. https://doi.org/10.2105/AJPH.2010.200915
5. Fowler MG, Johnson M, Atkinson S. School achievement and absence in children with chronic health conditions. *J Pediatr*. 1985;106(4): 683–687. https://doi.org/10.1016/S0022-3476(85)80103-7
6. Rethorn ZD, Cook C, Reneker JC. Social determinants of health: if you aren't measuring them, you aren't seeing the big picture. *J Orthop Sports Phys Ther*. 2019;49(12):872–874. https://doi.org/10.2519/jospt.2019.0613.
7. Degoy E, Olmos R. Reciprocal relation between health and academic performance in children through autoregressive models. *Sch Psychol*. 2020;35(5):332–342. https://doi.org/10.1037/spq0000409
8. Berkman ND, Sheridan SL, Donahue KE, Halpern DJ, Crotty K. Low health literacy and health outcomes: an updated systematic review. *Ann Intern Med*. 2011;155(2):97–107. https://doi.org/10.7326/0003-4819-155-2-201107190-00005
9. DeWalt DA, Hink A. Health literacy and child health outcomes: a systematic review of the literature. *Pediatrics*. 2009;124(suppl 3):S265–S274. https://doi.org/10.1542/peds.2009-1162B
10. Pignone M, DeWalt DA, Sheridan S, Berkman N, Lohr KN. Interventions to improve health outcomes for patients with low literacy. *J Gen Intern Med*. 2005;20(2):185–192. https://doi.org/10.1111/j.1525-1497.2005.40208.x
11. Jürges H, Reinhold S, Salm M. Does schooling affect health behavior? Evidence from the educational expansion in Western Germany. *Econ Educ Rev*. 2011;30(5):862–872. https://doi.org/10.1016/j.econedurev.2011.04.002
12. Hall PA, Fong GT. Temporal self-regulation theory: a model for individual health behavior. *Health Psychol Rev*. 2007;1(1):6–52. https://doi.org/10.1080/17437190701492437
13. Alakaam A, Lett M, Puckett H, Kite K. Associations among eating habits, health conditions, and education level in North Dakota adults. *Health Behav Policy Rev*. 2022;9(1):636–644. https://doi.org/10.14485/HBPR.9.1.2
14. Bratti M, Cottini E, Ghinetti P. Education, health and health-related behaviors: evidence from higher education expansion. January 2022. Available at: https://docs.iza.org/dp15035.pdf. Accessed June 23, 2024.
15. Hahn RA, Truman BI, Williams DR. Civil rights as determinants of public health and racial and ethnic health equity: health care, education, employment, and housing in the United States. *SSM Popul Health*. 2018;4:17–24. https://doi.org/10.1016/j.ssmph.2017.10.006
16. Paciência I, Cavaleiro Rufo J, Ribeiro AI, et al. Association between the density and type of trees around urban schools and exhaled nitric oxide levels in schoolchildren. *Eur Ann Allergy Clin Immunol*. 2021;53(1):29–36. https://doi.org/10.23822/EurAnnACI.1764-1489.162
17. Ryan CL, Bauman K. Educational attainment in the United States: 2015. March 29, 2016. Available at: https://www.census.gov/library/publications/2016/demo/p20-578.html. Accessed June 23, 2024.
18. Sullivan K, Thakur N. Structural and social determinants of health in asthma in developed economies: a scoping review of literature published between 2014 and 2019. *Curr Allergy Asthma Rep*. 2020;20(2):5. https://doi.org/10.1007/s11882-020-0899-6
19. Kivimäki M, Virtanen M, Kawachi I, et al. Long working hours, socioeconomic status, and the risk of incident type 2 diabetes: a meta-analysis of published and unpublished data from 222 120 individuals. *Lancet Diabetes Endocrinol*. 2015;3(1): 27–34. https://doi.org/10.1016/S2213-8587(14)70178-0
20. Mirowsky J, Ross CE. *Education, Social Status, and Health*. New York, NY: Routledge; 2017. https://doi.org/10.4324/9781351328081
21. Lynch J, Smith GD. A life course approach to chronic disease epidemiology. *Annu Rev Public Health*. 2005;26:1–35. https://doi.org/10.1146/annurev.publhealth.26.021304.144505
22. Berkman LF, Glass T. Social integration, social networks, social support, and health. In: Berkman LF, Kawachi I, eds. *Social Epidemiology*. New York, NY: Oxford Academic; 2000:137–173. https://doi.org/10.1093/oso/9780195083316.003.0007.
23. Hanushek EA, Peterson PE, Talpey LM, Woessmann L. The achievement gap fails to close. *Educ Next*. 2019;19(3):8–17.
24. Hanushek EA, Light JD, Peterson PE, Talpey LM, Woessmann L. Long-run trends in the US SES–achievement gap. *Educ Finance Policy*. 2022;17(4):608–640. https://doi.org/10.1162/edfp_a_00383
25. Chandra S, Chang A, Day L, et al. Closing the K–12 digital divide in the age of distance

learning. 2020. Available at: https://www.commonsensemedia.org/sites/default/files/research/report/common_sense_media_report_final_7_1_3pm_web.pdf. Accessed June 23, 2024.

26. Chalupka S, Anderko L. Climate change and schools: implications for children's health and safety. *Creat Nurs*. 2019;25(3):249–257. https://doi.org/10.1891/1078-4535.25.3.249
27. Baker R, Klasik D, Reardon SF. Race and stratification in college enrollment over time. *AERA Open*. 2018;4(1):2332858417751896. https://doi.org/10.1177/2332858417751896
28. Lee J. Racial and ethnic achievement gap trends: reversing the progress toward equity? *Educ Res*. 2002;31(1):3–12. https://doi.org/10.3102/0013189X031001003
29. Below A. Climate change: the existential threat multiplier. In: Gueldry M, Gokcek G, Hebron L, eds. *Understanding New Security Threats*. New York, NY: Routledge; 2019.
30. Sprague NL, Rundle AG, Ekenga CC. The COVID-19 pandemic as a threat multiplier for childhood health disparities: evidence from St. Louis, MO. *J Urban Health*. 2022;99(2):1–10. https://doi.org/10.1007/s11524-022-00616-8
31. Kimbro RT, Bzostek S, Goldman N, Rodríguez G. Race, ethnicity, and the education gradient in health. *Health Aff (Millwood)*. 2008;27(2):361–372. https://doi.org/10.1377/hlthaff.27.2.361
32. Nitardy CM, Duke NN, Pettingell SL, Borowsky IW. Racial and ethnic disparities in educational achievement and aspirations: findings from a statewide survey from 1998 to 2010. *Matern Child Health J*. 2015;19(1):58–66. https://doi.org/10.1007/s10995-014-1495-y
33. Hargrove TW, Gaydosh L, Dennis AC. Contextualizing educational disparities in health: variations by race/ethnicity, nativity, and county-level characteristics. *Demography*. 2022;59(1):267–292. https://doi.org/10.1215/00703370-9664206

Building Power on "Mass&Cass": A Community-Centered Approach to Addressing Health Resource Gaps for Persons Experiencing Homelessness in Boston, MA, 2021

Kareem I. King Jr, BA, Eileen Milien, BS, Melissa Jones, Terrance Mensah, BA, MPhil, MD, and Lady Lawrence E.J. Carty, AB

In November 2021, two grassroots organizations in Boston, Massachusetts—a housing and health justice organization and a student-led nonprofit—established an initiative to provide persons experiencing homelessness (PEH) near the Massachusetts Avenue and Melnea Cass Boulevard ("Mass&Cass") intersection in Boston with access to free COVID-19 education and other wrap-around services. They partnered with hospitals, public health organizations, and advocacy groups to make this happen. This community-driven initiative serves as a model for how to enact a sustainable pipeline for PEH to receive health resources and information, with the voices of those directly impacted at the center. (*Am J Public Health*. 2024;114(9):870–873. https://doi.org/10.2105/AJPH.2024.307713)

AJPH September 2024, Vol. 114, No. 9

The COVID-19 pandemic highlighted historic structural inequities in both health care and resource provision that have existed in underserved communities for decades.[1] Persons experiencing homelessness (PEH) are among the most underserved populations.

INTERVENTION AND IMPLEMENTATION

The goals of this joint project with the Rapid Acceleration of Diagnostics–Underserved Populations (RADx-UP) Initiative were to (1) take direction from affected communities to address their most acute needs, (2) empower them with accurate health information and resources to mitigate COVID-19 transmission during the pandemic, and (3) show that community support is a model for engaging unhoused people in stable access to health care services and resources.

As part of the community support model, our organizations—Housing = Health, a housing and health justice initiative, and We Got Us, a student-led nonprofit focused on health equity—came together to provide COVID-19 resources and other wrap-around services at four sites in Boston, Massachusetts on a biweekly basis. These locations were chosen by community members, in consultation with the Boston Health Care for the Homeless Program (BHCHP), a local federally qualified health center, based on where the most pressing needs were. Community members had equal decision-making power in determining the budget for this initiative and resource allocation.

At each location, an outreach table was set up to provide PEH with information on COVID-19 vaccination, testing, and other resources (Table 1). Each quarter, resources changed to meet emerging needs voiced by the community. For example, in the late spring, summer, and fall months (quarters 1 and 2), we provided items such as sunscreen and rain ponchos. However, quarters 3 and 4 fell during the winter and early spring months, so we adapted our resource kits to include winter survival items (hats, gloves, scarves, blankets, and hand warmers). Those who had acute care needs were directed to the BHCHP. This program was driven by community members with lived experience in being

TABLE 1— Number of Resource Kits Distributed, by Quarter: Boston, Massachusetts, April 1, 2022–March 31, 2023

Quarter	No. of Resource Kits Distributed	Quarter-Specific Materials	All Quarters
1	842	Sunscreen, rain ponchos, prepackaged food	N95 masks, surgical masks, hand sanitizer, COVID-19 tests, water bottles, soap, toothbrushes, toothpaste, granola bars, tote bags, nitrile gloves, debit cards
2	496		
3	782	Winter gloves, scarves, hats, socks, hand wipes, handwarmers, prepackaged food	
4	438	Winter gloves, scarves, hats, socks, hand wipes, handwarmers, coats, blankets, winter clothing	
Total	2558	...	...

unhoused, to ensure the services provided were most in line with the needs being expressed.

PLACE, TIME, AND PERSONS

This project started in November 2021. We partnered with the BHCHP to serve as COVID-19 ambassadors for PEH near the Massachusetts Avenue and Melnea Cass Boulevard ("Mass&Cass") intersection in Boston, Massachusetts. The BHCHP treats roughly 11 000 unhoused people each year.[2] This population experiences an increased burden of substance use disorder, mental illness, and HIV, among other health risks, because of the realities of being unhoused.[3] This article describes the intervention's results from April 2022 to March 2023.

PURPOSE

PEH in the United States are 6 to 10 times more likely to have unmet medical needs than the general population.[4] Furthermore, the harsh conditions faced by unhoused people put them at increased risk for COVID-19 infection and death.[5] Our goal was to create an initiative that addresses the unique health needs of unhoused people in Boston, utilizing a community support model.

At the height of the pandemic (2020–2021), public health guidelines noted social distancing, proper mask wearing, and getting the COVID-19 vaccine as key measures for reducing COVID-19 spread. City guidelines that were put in place to limit disease spread could not be completely followed in shelters, because of severe space constraints.

Organizations at the local and state level took action to attempt to mitigate the impact on PEH. In 2021, the Massachusetts Legislature's Health Equity Task Force released a report that recommended providing hotel or motel rooms for unhoused people along with guidelines for funding it, using federal monies awarded to the state to respond to the pandemic.[6] In the same year, Housing = Health worked with state representatives to propose a $5 million budget request for unhoused people to be provided with smartphones for telehealth, which was ultimately denied.

This trend speaks to a larger pattern of injustice and neglect for the unique health needs of unhoused people. When the COVID-19 vaccine first rolled out in December 2020, people aged 65 years and older and those with comorbidities were among the earliest groups eligible to receive the shot. In most states, unhoused people were not on the list of those prioritized, even though their likelihood of possessing underlying comorbidities is higher than in the general population.[7,8] This drove us to develop a new initiative that centered those needs at the outset.

EVALUATION AND ADVERSE EFFECTS

From April 2022 to March 2023, we hosted 28 outreach events and had more than 3000 interactions at our table. We provided PEH with COVID-19 information and over 2558 resource kits (Figure 1). By having a consistent presence, we were able to build rapport with the persons who regularly visited our table and become a trusted source of information.

This initiative included built-in feedback pathways to incorporate the community voice into our work. At each event, individuals were asked to complete a voluntary survey to gauge vaccination status and asked whether they had a smartphone that they could use to access telehealth services; 500 people completed this survey. This served to engage PEH in conversations about the barriers they were facing to

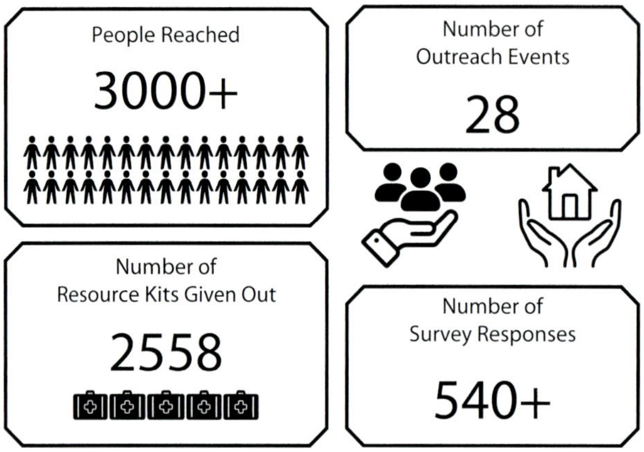

FIGURE 1— Data Showing Overall Impact of the Project: Boston, Massachusetts, April 1, 2022–March 31, 2023

receiving the vaccine or other health care services and update them on current public health guidelines (such as changing regulations on masking in indoor vs outdoor spaces). This data also provided a pathway for us to translate what we learned back to our institutional partners through regular check-ins.

In addition to the brief survey, PEH were invited to participate in longer interviews with our research team to discuss their experience utilizing our program and improvements they would like to see in their ability to access care; 40 people completed this interview. Although many individuals reported that they had places they could visit to receive care (e.g., BHCHP clinics, shelters, emergency rooms), distance was noted as a significant barrier for this access. Providing a smartphone for telehealth was intended to help overcome this barrier.

Some of the major challenges we faced included resource constraints as emergency funding dissipated for COVID-19 relief projects, changing city guidelines on the kinds of resources community groups were able to provide to PEH, and gaining support from a medical center to implement a telehealth initiative specifically for unhoused people. With the help of our partner organizations, we were able to address most of these challenges. Furthermore, we created the infrastructure needed to start our telehealth initiative in the summer of 2023, a method that has been shown to positively affect connection to health care for unhoused individuals.[9,10]

SUSTAINABILITY

This initiative was driven by a coalition of local nonprofit organizations, health advocacy groups, and students (high school, college, and graduate level) located in Boston. We Got Us boasts a network of students from minoritized backgrounds dedicated to providing accurate health information to underresourced communities.[11] Housing = Health, a health advocacy organization whose founder and executive director has over 30 years of experience operating in the housing advocacy space, has significant ties to the local community and understands the needs that currently exist. By leveraging our partnerships with the various hospitals, national organizations, and health centers we connected with over our project year, this initiative is continuing strong, and expanding to incorporate telehealth as an additional service within our community support model.

PUBLIC HEALTH SIGNIFICANCE

The COVID-19 pandemic highlighted the health inequities that PEH face, and our model provided the necessary infrastructure to support public health measures and build rapport for future health emergencies. Through our joint initiative, we were able to provide consistent public health resources to unhoused people, break accessibility barriers to COVID-19–related information, and establish a bidirectional pipeline of trusted public health messaging that spans hospitals, nonprofits, and public health institutions. This project also provided us with the platform we needed for subsequent efforts to connect PEH with stable access to health care services, through telehealth. Moreover, it demonstrated the value of empowering those most impacted by health disparities to drive public health relief efforts in their own communities. AJPH

ABOUT THE AUTHORS

Kareem I. King Jr. and Melissa Jones are with We Got Us, Boston, MA, and Harvard College, Cambridge, MA. Eilien Milien is with We Got Us, Boston, and

Emmanuel College, Boston. Terrence Mensah is with Housing = Health, Boston, and Harvard Medical School, Boston. Lady Lawrence E. J. Carty is with Housing = Health, Boston.

CORRESPONDENCE

Correspondence should be sent to Kareem King at 72 East Concord Street, Evans Building, Floor 7, Boston, MA 02118 (e-mail: k.kingi2023@gmail.com). Reprints can be ordered at https://www.ajph.org by clicking the "Reprints" link.

PUBLICATION INFORMATION

Full Citation: King KI Jr, Milien E, Jones M, Mensah T, Carty LLEJ. Building power on "Mass&Cass": a community-centered approach to addressing health resource gaps for persons experiencing homelessness in Boston, MA, 2021. *Am J Public Health*. 2024;114(9):870–873.

Acceptance Date: April 21, 2024.

DOI: https://doi.org/10.2105/AJPH.2024.307713

ORCID iD:

Kareem I. King https://orcid.org/0000-0002-7025-4618

CONTRIBUTORS

All authors contributed to the conceptualization, drafting, and revising of the manuscript, as well as physical participation in the outreach initiative detailed. K. I. King Jr., E. Milien, and L. L. E. J. Carty secured funding. All authors approved the final version of the manuscript.

ACKNOWLEDGMENTS

Findings reported in this Rapid Acceleration of Diagnostics–Underserved Populations (RADx-UP) publication was supported by the National Institutes of Health (award no. C0437).

We thank the following individuals and organizations who were critical in allowing us to do this work: Jessie Gaeta and Denise de las Nueces from Boston Health Care for the Homeless Program; Bisola Ojikutu and Gerry Thomas from the Boston Public Health Commission; Dwayne Brown from Southampton Men's Shelter; and Paul Johnson and Savina Martin from the Massachusetts Union of the Homeless. We also appreciate the various staff and volunteers who contributed directly to helping sustain our outreach initiative: Taina Rico, Giovanni Monteiro Do Canto, Jemel Bates, Marc-Kendy Paul, Dominick Contreras, Sarah Koolsbergen, and many others who could not be listed. Special thanks to LaShyra Nolen, the founder and executive director of We Got Us, for hosting and supporting this initiative and Regina LaRocque from Massachusetts General Hospital for guiding the submission of our RADx-UP project grant and serving as a trusted advisor throughout the process.

Note. The contents are solely the responsibility of the authors and do not necessarily represent the official views of the National Institutes of Health.

CONFLICTS OF INTEREST

The authors report that there are no competing interests to declare.

HUMAN PARTICIPANT PROTECTION

The data we collected were not used in the formation of a research study, and therefore institutional review board approval was not required. All data were anonymous and do not include personal identifiers.

REFERENCES

1. Ndugga N, Artiga S. Disparities in health and health care: 5 key questions and answers. Kaiser Family Foundation. May 11, 2021. Available at: https://www.kff.org/racial-equity-and-health-policy/issue-brief/disparities-in-health-and-health-care-5-key-question-and-answers. Accessed January 29, 2023.
2. Boston Health Care for the Homeless Program. Building telehealth and behavioral health programs during pandemic. *The View From the Bridge*. Fall 2020. Available at: https://www.bhchp.org/wp-content/uploads/2022/12/FINAL-copy_digital.pdf. Accessed January 29, 2023.
3. Baggett TP, Hwang SW, O'Connell JJ, et al. Mortality among homeless adults in Boston. *JAMA Intern Med*. 2013;173(3):189–195. https://doi.org/10.1001/jamainternmed.2013.1604
4. Fleury MJ, Grenier G, Sabetti J, Bertrand K, Clément M, Brochu S. Met and unmet needs of homeless individuals at different stages of housing reintegration: a mixed-method investigation. *PLoS One*. 2021;16(1):e0245088. https://doi.org/10.1371/journal.pone.0245088
5. Perri M, Dosani N, Hwang SW. COVID-19 and people experiencing homelessness: challenges and mitigation strategies. *CMAJ*. 2020;192(26):E716–E719. https://doi.org/10.1503/cmaj.200834
6. The 193rd General Court of the Commonwealth of Massachusetts. Health Equity Task Force. Health Equity Task Force final report—a blueprint for health equity. Available at: https://malegislature.gov/Commissions/Detail/512/Documents. Accessed January 30, 2023.
7. Trick WE, Rachman F, Hinami K, et al. Variability in comorbidities and health services use across homeless typologies: multicenter data linkage between healthcare and homeless systems. *BMC Public Health*. 2021;21(1):917. https://doi.org/10.1186/s12889-021-10958-8
8. Van Ness L. States fail to prioritize homeless people for vaccines. *Stateline*. March 1, 2021. Available at: https://www.pewtrusts.org/en/research-and-analysis/blogs/stateline/2021/03/01/states-fail-to-prioritize-homeless-people-for-vaccines. Accessed January 30, 2023.
9. Adams CS, Player MS, Berini CR, et al. A telehealth initiative to overcome health care barriers for people experiencing homelessness. *Telemed J E Health*. 2021;27(8):851–858. https://doi.org/10.1089/tmj.2021.0127
10. Kazevman G, Mercado M, Hulme J, Somers A. Prescribing phones to address health equity needs in the COVID-19 era: The PHONE-CONNECT Program. *J Med Internet Res*. 2021;23(4):e23914. https://doi.org/10.2196/23914
11. Milien E, Enoma E, Pierre-Louis L, et al. We Got Us: A community-centered approach to increasing vaccine access for minoritized groups. *J Hosp Med*. 2022;17(9):765–768. https://doi.org/10.1002/jhm.12927

Scaling Emergency Department Opioid Use Disorder Treatment Across California to Reduce Overdose Deaths, 2019–2023

Elizabeth A. Samuels, MD, MPH, MHS, Allison D. Rosen, PhD, Melissa Speener, MPH, John Kaleekal, MPH, MBA, Mariah M. Kalmin, PhD, MHS, David Goodman-Meza, MD, Steve Shoptaw, PhD, Serena Clayton, PhD, Chunqing Lin, PhD, Arianna Campbell, PA-C, Aimee Moulin, MD, and Andrew A. Herring, MD

Since April 2019, CA Bridge has worked with emergency departments (EDs) in diverse geographic and emergency care settings across California to scale up low-threshold buprenorphine access, patient navigation programs, harm reduction services, and take-home naloxone. Between April 2019 and June 2023, 268 (81.0%) of 331 acute care hospitals in California received funding and technical assistance from CA Bridge and completed data reporting. These hospitals provided navigation services during 279 025 patient encounters and gave patients buprenorphine in 89 549 ED visits. (*Am J Public Health*. 2024;114(9):874–878. https://doi.org/10.2105/AJPH.2024.307710)

AJPH September 2024, Vol. 114, No. 9

The emergency department (ED) is a critical site for the delivery of evidence-based harm reduction and addiction treatment to reduce overdose deaths.[1] Buprenorphine is an opioid agonist medication that reduces both all-cause and overdose mortality among people with opioid use disorder (OUD).[2,3] ED buprenorphine initiation for the treatment of OUD is safe[4,5] and can improve outpatient treatment linkage.[6] ED naloxone distribution is feasible and acceptable.[7] Furthermore, patient navigation for ED patients with OUD can improve engagement in outpatient services.[8] Many ED OUD treatment and harm reduction programs are implemented in response to state or local regulations[9] or financial incentives,[10] or are supported by local, state, or federal grants.[11] The largest statewide incentivized ED buprenorphine initiative is CA Bridge in California.

INTERVENTION AND IMPLEMENTATION

In 2016, CA Bridge began as a pilot initiative (ED Bridge) supported by the California Health Care Foundation to improve emergency care for individuals with OUD using a model with three core elements: rapid access to low-barrier buprenorphine, navigation to outpatient care, and harm reduction. With additional support from the Public Health Institute, CA Bridge expanded across California, providing training, technical assistance, and financial support to deliver evidence-based ED OUD care.

Hospitals participating in CA Bridge were provided funding to initiate or expand the CA Bridge model within their ED. Funding supported a local clinical champion and a patient navigator to provide ED patients with harm reduction and addiction treatment services, including buprenorphine treatment of OUD, take-home naloxone, and linkage to outpatient care (BridgeToTreatment.org). Patient navigators engaged patients at the time of their ED visit and worked with clinicians to provide ED-administered buprenorphine and buprenorphine prescriptions, take-home naloxone, harm reduction education, and linkage to outpatient addiction treatment. Linkage included scheduling appointments, follow-up phone calls with patients, and transportation arrangement. The harm reduction services provided varied by site, and included provision of take-home naloxone, fentanyl test strips, and overdose prevention education. Hospital champions and navigators were advised through clinical guidelines, trainings, site visits, educational webinars, and real-time implementation support from CA Bridge staff. Participating sites reported information about implementation milestones and aggregate data about patients and ED services on a quarterly basis.

PLACE, TIME, AND PERSONS

California has 331 acute care hospitals serving 39.24 million people in rural, suburban, and urban areas.[12] Among these, 56 are designated public or district municipal public hospitals, 22 are academic medical centers, and 36 are critical access hospitals.[13] CA Bridge was scaled across California from April 2019 through June 2023 through three successive funding rounds. All California hospitals were eligible to apply for funding. Hospitals were eligible to reapply for continued funding at the end of each round. In the first round (April 2019–September 2020), an initial cohort of 52 hospitals was supported by State Opioid Response funding. From October 2020 to June 2022, a second round of 200 hospitals was supported through the California Department of Health Care Services (DHCS)-funded Behavioral Health Pilot Project (75.5% newly funded). In the third round (July 2022–June 2023), 241 hospitals were supported with funds from the California DHCS authorized by the American Rescue Plan Act of 2021 (27% newly funded; Figures 1 and 2).

The present evaluation includes all ED encounters where a patient was seen for a substance use disorder between April 2019 and June 2023 at any of 268 participating hospitals that implemented the CA Bridge model and completed data-reporting requirements.

PURPOSE

California is the most populous state in the United States. In 2021, more than 10 898 Californians died of an opioid overdose, with a death rate of 26.6 deaths per 100 000 people.[14] CA Bridge is the primary state-supported effort to expand ED OUD treatment. Nearly all California hospitals (81.0%; 268/331) applied for and received funding and technical assistance through CA Bridge and reported data in at least one funding round. Whereas prior work described initial implementation efforts over the first 14 months of the program,[11] this analysis assessed

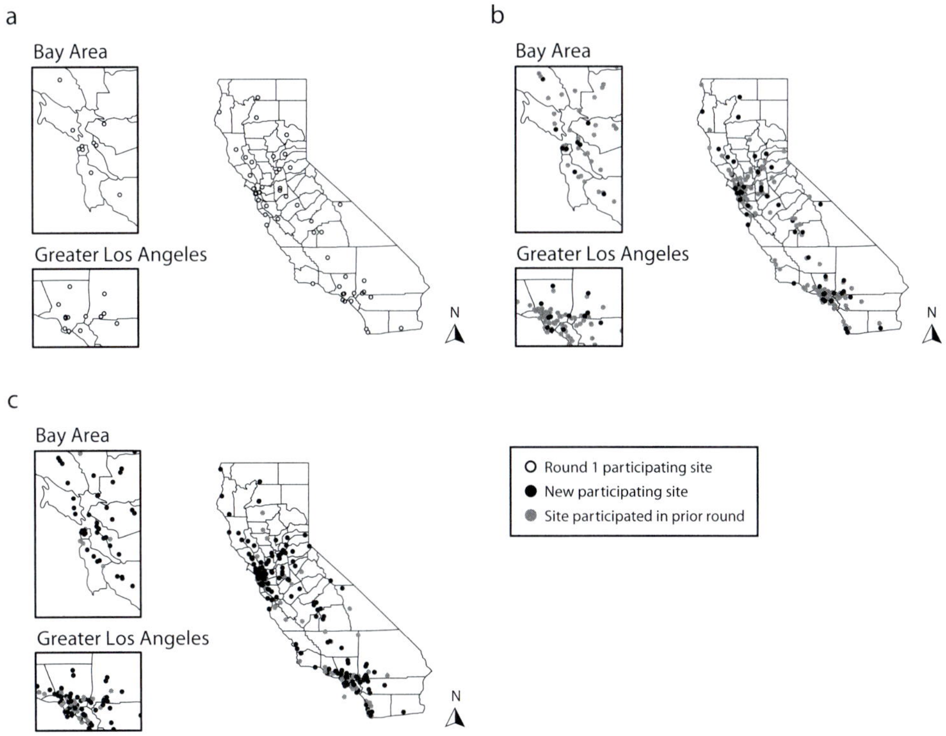

FIGURE 1— Locations of CA Bridge–Participating Hospitals in (a) First, (b) Second, and (c) Third Funding Rounds: California, April 2019–June 2023

Note. Shown are hospitals in each funding round that completed data reporting. The first funding round (April 2019–September 2020) reached 15.7% (52/331) of California hospitals, the second (October 2020–June 2022) reached 60.4% (200/331), and the third (July 2022–June 2023) reached 72.8% (241/331). A total of 268 unique hospitals participated in at least one funding round and completed data reporting, reaching 81.0% of California hospitals.

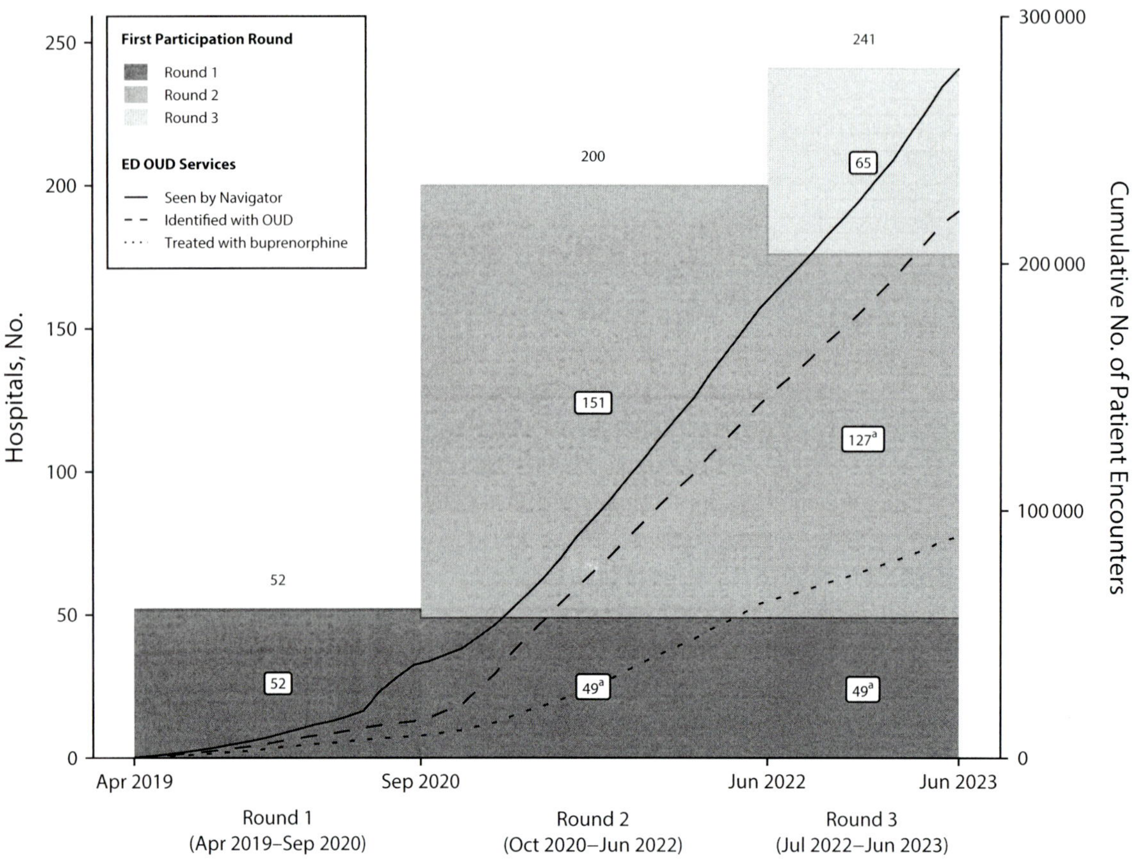

FIGURE 2— CA Bridge–Participating Hospitals and Services Provided, by Funding Round: California, April 2019–June 2023

Note. ED = emergency department; OUD = opioid use disorder. Shown are CA Bridge–participating hospitals and encounters where patients were seen by a patient navigator, identified with opioid use disorder, and administered or prescribed buprenorphine.
[a]Not all hospitals that participated in one round participated in the following round(s).The first funding round was April 2019 to September 2020, second was October 2020 to June 2022, and the third was July 2022 through June 2023.

the scaling of CA Bridge implementation across California.

EVALUATION AND ADVERSE EFFECTS

We evaluated monthly hospital-reported data in aggregate as proportions, counts, and summary statistics. The median number of patients seen by navigators, identified with OUD, and administered or prescribed buprenorphine across hospitals was calculated for the first and last month of data reporting. Changes between the first and last month were assessed using a Wilcoxon Signed-Rank Test.

Hospitals reported data for a median 29 months (interquartile range [IQR] = 12–32). In the first implementation round at 52 hospitals, patient navigators were consulted during 35 905 encounters, OUD was identified at 14 432 encounters, and buprenorphine treatment (ED administration or discharge prescription) was provided at 8743 encounters (Figure 2). During the second round, when the program expanded to 200 hospitals, we observed increases in encounters with navigator consultation (n = 146 480), OUD identification (n = 128 891), and buprenorphine treatment (n = 53 791). During the third round, expansion to 241 hospitals resulted in an additional 96 640 navigator consults, 77 922 patient encounters where OUD was identified, and 27 015 encounters where buprenorphine treatment was provided. Across the 268 unique hospitals from all three rounds, patient navigators were consulted in 279 025 ED encounters, OUD was identified in 221 245 encounters, and buprenorphine treatment was provided in 89 549 encounters (Figure 2).

During their first month of implementation regardless of funding round, hospitals reported a median of 0 (IQR = 0–1; range = 0–228) navigator encounters, 7 (IQR = 1–24;

range = 0–258) patients identified with OUD, and 1 (IQR = 0–5; range = 0–80) encounter where buprenorphine was administered or prescribed. By their final month of data reporting, hospitals reported a median of 24 (IQR = 6–58; range = 0–464) navigator encounters ($P < .001$), 15 (IQR = 6–39; range 0–313) patients identified with OUD ($P < .001$), and 5 (IQR = 1–15; range 0–167) encounters where buprenorphine was administered or prescribed ($P < .001$). Provision of services was highest at EDs with higher annual patient volumes (Table A, available as a supplement to the online version of this article at http://www.ajph.org).

SUSTAINABILITY

CA Bridge implementation was supported by funding provided directly to hospitals. Among the 203 hospitals participating in the first two funding rounds, the majority (n = 176; 86.7%) reapplied for funding in the subsequent round to continue their program. This suggests that participating hospitals valued their program, opting to continue to work with CA Bridge and provide ED buprenorphine, patient navigation, and harm reduction services to ED patients with OUD.

Although CA Bridge succeeded in initial reach and scale-up to bring OUD treatment to most California EDs, there is a need for additional work to support program financial sustainability, improve implementation, and integrate the ED into the continuum of substance use disorder care. Like initiatives in other states, CA Bridge has been funded by time-limited, state-based opioid response grants. California has taken several steps to support financial sustainability for patient navigator and ED OUD services. Under Medi-Cal, California's Medicaid program, hospitals may bill for community health worker services. This is an important advancement; without sufficient patient volumes, however, reimbursement rates may not sustainably support full-time staffing.

Despite success at engaging a wide variety of hospitals, there was significant variability in services delivery, with a broad range of extremely high-performing and low-performing sites, despite equivalent and significant resources provided to participating sites. Further work is needed to improve implementation and services delivery at lower-performing sites and identify and incentivize high-quality care. With the groundwork laid by CA Bridge to engage hospitals and establish treatment protocols, quality performance initiatives may be effective tools to enhance services delivery. The California DHCS has established a quality incentive pool to improve ED addiction care at public institutions. The Healthcare Effectiveness Data and Information Set has quality performance incentives for outpatient addiction treatment follow-up seven and 30 days after a substance use–related ED visit. Both of these performance reimbursement strategies could be leveraged to improve emergency addiction care delivery.

Participating sites are working to sustain their navigators; however, additional initiatives at the county, state, and federal levels are needed to sustain emergency addiction care. Altogether, 80.5% of participating sites (194/241) have either sustained, or are in the process of working to sustain, their patient navigator. Currently, 35.7% (86/241) of CA Bridge hospitals funded in round 3 have reported successfully sustaining their patient navigator outside of CA Bridge–related grant funding. An additional 108 sites (44.8%) are in the process of making the position permanent. Although this is an important and meaningful start to maintaining current patient navigation services among CA Bridge hospitals, many hospitals are at risk for losing their programs without future funding. To maintain patient navigators who facilitate the delivery of high-quality care to patients with OUD, reimbursements and quality performance incentives are needed at state and national levels to ensure adequate funding of these essential ED services.

PUBLIC HEALTH SIGNIFICANCE

The CA Bridge model bundles three primary evidenced-based interventions for ED patients with OUD—low-threshold buprenorphine, harm reduction, and linkage to long-term outpatient care through patient navigation. The rapid, successful scale-up of CA Bridge across California suggests that this is a promising implementation model for dissemination to other states to expand low-threshold addiction treatment access as part of a national strategy to address the overdose crisis. AJPH

ABOUT THE AUTHORS

Elizabeth A. Samuels is with the Department of Emergency Medicine, Allison D. Rosen and Steve Shoptaw are with the Department of Family Medicine, and David Goodman-Meza is with the Division of Infectious Diseases, David Geffen School of Medicine, University of California, Los Angeles. Melissa Speener, John Kaleekal, Serena Clayton, Arianna Campbell, and Andrew A. Herring are with CA Bridge, Public Health Institute, Oakland, CA. Mariah M. Kalmin is with the RAND Corporation, Santa Monica, CA. Chunqing Lin is with the Department of Psychiatry and Biobehavioral Sciences, University of California, Los Angeles. Aimee Moulin is with the Marshall Medical Center, Placerville, CA.

CORRESPONDENCE

Correspondence should be sent to Elizabeth A. Samuels, MD, MPH, MHS, Department of Emergency Medicine, David Geffen School of Medicine, University of California, Los Angeles, 1100 Glendon Ave, Suite 1200, Los Angeles, CA 90024 (e-mail: lizsamuels@ucla.edu). Reprints can be ordered at https://www.ajph.org by clicking the "Reprints" link.

PUBLICATION INFORMATION

Full Citation: Samuels EA, Rosen AD, Speener M, et al. Scaling emergency department opioid use disorder treatment across California to reduce overdose deaths, 2019–2023. *Am J Public Health*. 2024;114(9):874–878.

Acceptance Date: April 21, 2024.

DOI: https://doi.org/10.2105/AJPH.2024.307710

ORCID iDs:

Elizabeth A. Samuels https://orcid.org/0000-0003-2414-110X

Allison D. Rosen https://orcid.org/0000-0002-1630-0222

CONTRIBUTORS

E. A. Samuels, A. D. Rosen, M. Speener, J. Kaleekal, M. M. Kalmin, D. Goodman-Meza, S. Shoptaw, C. Lin, and A. A. Herring conceptualized the manuscript. A. D. Rosen conducted data analysis with supervision from E. A. Samuels and M. M. Kalmin. A. D. Rosen, D. Goodman-Meza, and E. A. Samuels developed manuscript figures. E. A. Samuels and A. D. Rosen drafted the manuscript. All authors contributed substantively to manuscript revision. E. A. Samuels takes responsibility for the manuscript as a whole.

ACKNOWLEDGMENTS

E. A. Samuels is partially supported by the Centers for Disease Control and Prevention (R01CE003632).

We thank the CA Bridge program and administrative teams and CA Bridge-participating hospital clinical site champions and patient navigators for their tireless work to improve the health of people with substance use disorders.

Note. The authors assume full responsibility for the accuracy and completeness of the ideas presented, which do not represent the views of the Centers for Disease Control and Prevention, the Public Health Institute, the RAND Corporation, or any other supporting institutions.

CONFLICTS OF INTEREST

The co-authors include co-founders of CA Bridge and CA Bridge staff. The authors have no financial conflicts of interest to disclose.

HUMAN PARTICIPANT PROTECTION

This is a retrospective evaluation of aggregate, de-identified administrative data from a public health program, and is exempt from institutional review board review.

REFERENCES

1. Vivolo-Kantor AM, Seth P, Gladden RM, et al. Vital signs: trends in emergency department visits for suspected opioid overdoses—United States, July 2016–September 2017. *MMWR Morb Mortal Wkly Rep*. 2018;67(9):279–285. https://doi.org/10.15585/mmwr.mm6709e1
2. Santo T Jr, Clark B, Hickman M, et al. Association of opioid agonist treatment with all-cause mortality and specific causes of death among people with opioid dependence: a systematic review and meta-analysis. *JAMA Psychiatry*. 2021;78(9):979–993. https://doi.org/10.1001/jamapsychiatry.2021.0976
3. Sordo L, Barrio G, Bravo MJ, et al. Mortality risk during and after opioid substitution treatment: systematic review and meta-analysis of cohort studies. *BMJ*. 2017;357:j1550. https://doi.org/10.1136/bmj.j1550
4. Herring AA, Vosooghi AA, Luftig J, et al. High-dose buprenorphine induction in the emergency department for treatment of opioid use disorder. *JAMA Netw Open*. 2021;4(7):e2117128. https://doi.org/10.1001/jamanetworkopen.2021.17128
5. D'Onofrio G, Hawk KF, Perrone J, et al. Incidence of precipitated withdrawal during a multisite emergency department-initiated buprenorphine clinical trial in the era of fentanyl. *JAMA Netw Open*. 2023;6(3):e236108. https://doi.org/10.1001/jamanetworkopen.2023.6108
6. D'Onofrio G, O'Connor PG, Pantalon MV, et al. Emergency department-initiated buprenorphine/naloxone treatment for opioid dependence: a randomized clinical trial. *JAMA*. 2015;313(16):1636–1644. https://doi.org/10.1001/jama.2015.3474
7. Samuels EA, Baird J, Yang ES, Mello M. Adoption and utilization of an emergency department naloxone distribution and peer recovery coach consultation program. *Acad Emerg Med*. 2019;26(2):160–173.
8. Anderson ES, Rusoja E, Luftig J, et al. Effectiveness of substance use navigation for emergency department patients with substance use disorders: an implementation study. *Ann Emerg Med*. 2023;81(3):297–308. https://doi.org/10.1016/j.annemergmed.2022.09.025
9. Samuels EA, Wentz A, McCormick M, et al. Rhode Island's opioid overdose hospital standards and emergency department naloxone distribution, behavioral counseling, and referral to treatment. *Ann Emerg Med*. 2021;78(1):68–79. https://doi.org/10.1016/j.annemergmed.2021.02.004
10. Kilaru AS, Perrone J, Kelley D, et al. Participation in a hospital incentive program for follow-up treatment for opioid use disorder. *JAMA Netw Open*. 2020;3(1):e1918511. https://doi.org/10.1001/jamanetworkopen.2019.18511
11. Snyder H, Kalmin MM, Moulin A, et al. Rapid adoption of low-threshold buprenorphine treatment at California emergency departments participating in the CA Bridge Program. *Ann Emerg Med*. 2021;78(6):759–772. https://doi.org/10.1016/j.annemergmed.2021.05.024
12. California Health Care Foundation. California hospitals and emergency departments–almanac collection. July 2022. Available at: https://www.chcf.org/wp-content/uploads/2022/07/CAHospitalsAlmanac2022QRG.pdf. Accessed September 2023.
13. California Dept of Health Care Access and Information. Emergency department encounters. September 1, 2022. Available at: https://hcai.ca.gov. Accessed April 2023.
14. National Center for Health Statistics. Drug overdose mortality by state. 2022. Available at: https://www.cdc.gov/nchs/pressroom/sosmap/drug_poisoning_mortality/drug_poisoning.htm. Accessed April 2023.

Political Determinants of Health: Has COVID-19 Exposed the Worst of It?

Gerardo Chowell, PhD, and Nazrul Islam, MD, PhD

ABOUT THE AUTHORS

Gerardo Chowell is with the Department of Population Health Sciences, Georgia State University School of Public Health, Atlanta, and the Centre for Research on Pandemics and Society, Oslo Metropolitan University, Oslo, Norway. Nazrul Islam is with the Faculty of Medicine, University of Southampton, Southampton, UK, and the Max Planck Institute for Demographic Research, Rostock, Germany.

See also Woolf et al., p. 882.

The COVID-19 pandemic has underscored the deep connection between public health and political partisanship in the United States. The study by Woolf et al. in this issue of *AJPH* (p. 882) highlights significant differences in excess death rates across states and points to a troubling link between political leanings and mortality rates. The authors found that the states led by Republican governors and those with greater Republican representation experienced higher excess death rates during critical periods of the pandemic, highlighting the need to prioritize evidence-based decision-making over political considerations.

POLITICS, POLITICAL PARTISANSHIP, AND PANDEMIC RESPONSE

The findings align with those from the book *Pandemic Politics: The Deadly Toll of Partisanship in the Age of COVID* by Gadarian et al.,[1] which further supports the impact of political polarization on public health outcomes. On the basis of six public opinion surveys from March 2020 to April 2021, Gadarian et al. found that Democrats exhibited more prohealth behaviors, such as hand washing and mask wearing, than Republicans. Overall, the evidence emphasizes the real-life impact of political decisions on policies and people's lives. An urgent need exists for a united, nonpartisan, evidence-based approach to managing public health crises that goes beyond political divides and prioritizes the well-being of all citizens with a health equity lens.

POLITICAL INFLUENCE AND EXCESS DEATHS

The research of Woolf et al. on excess death rates during the COVID-19 pandemic adds to the body of work linking political partisanship and mortality impact across the United States. The study reveals that the United States experienced an estimated 1 277 697 excess deaths from March 2020 to July 2023. States led by Republican governors and those with greater Republican representation saw higher excess death rates, especially during the prevaccine and early vaccine phases. According to the study, compared with those led by Democratic governors, excess death was 64.5 per 100 000 population higher in the states led by Republican governors across the five phases of the pandemic.

This pattern highlights how political decisions directly impacted public health, as Republican-led states were less likely to implement preventive public health and social measures (also known as nonpharmaceutical interventions) such as face masks and physical distancing,[2–4] likely leading to higher mortality rates. Extensive literature on political and ideological differences noted that, compared with the liberal or Democratic views, conservative or Republican ideology is less responsive to radical policy measures with critical impact on personal autonomy (i.e., policies that challenge the "status quo") and economic growth.[5] Conservative views and beliefs might have led to prioritizing personal autonomy over collective altruism and resilience and the potential economic growth over human lives. Similar patterns of differential adoption of public health policies by political partisanship and their impact on COVID-19 morbidity and mortality were reported elsewhere, such as in Brazil.[6,7] While the study relied on widely used statistical modeling methods, the authors acknowledged the potential influence of confounding variables such as age distribution, racial/ethnic composition, and socioeconomic status, which were not fully adjusted for. These factors have been shown to have differential impacts on morbidity and

AJPH September 2024, Vol. 114, No. 9

mortality associated with the COVID-19 pandemic.[8–11]

The report by Woolf et al. provides valuable data on excess deaths in the United States overall and by state, which could benefit from including the uncertainties around the estimates, such as 95% confidence intervals. The study also revealed that more than half of the excess deaths occurred after vaccines became widely available, pointing to the impact of political partisanship on vaccine uptake and public health compliance. A cautious interpretation of these findings is required because the study was not designed to estimate the effect of COVID-19 vaccination on excess deaths. The analysis reported the excess deaths by the timeline of vaccine availability without taking into account the uptake of the vaccines. There was substantial variability across the states regarding COVID-19 vaccine coverage, speed, and uptake. Moreover, background COVID-19 infection rate, uptake, and adherence to nonpharmaceutical interventions also varied substantially by state. Lastly, even though the study does not measure the direct causal effect of political ideology on excess deaths, it clearly provides the differential impacts of the estimated causal effect of the pandemic and associated policy measures on excess deaths by political partisanship at the individual and policy levels. This is a critical contribution of the study.

Integrating findings from the study by Woolf et al. on excess death rates with insights from the work of others paints a clearer picture of how political partisanship shaped the public health landscape during the COVID-19 pandemic.[1,12] Collectively, these findings portray how the fragmented response to COVID-19 exacerbated the pandemic's toll and deepened societal inequities. Looking ahead, fostering bipartisan cooperation and strictly adhering to scientific guidelines will be essential in mitigating the impacts of future public health emergencies. These insights support the case for policy reforms to bridge the partisan divide and safeguard public health. This can be achieved through transparent communication, consistent policies across political lines, and robust public health education campaigns prioritizing facts over politics.[12,13] There are hundreds of societal and policy examples jointly supported by the Republicans and Democrats (e.g., Social Security, affordable housing, prekindergarten education). Therefore, a bipartisan pandemic preparedness roadmap could be agreed upon highlighting the nuances of critical issues of differences such as personal autonomy during a pandemic or similar health emergencies (e.g., highlighting the greater societal altruism and resilience, and its potential beneficial effects on at-risk populations, such as the elderly and those with underlying chronic diseases) and prioritizing human lives over economic growth.

The COVID-19 pandemic has had a profound toll on human lives. Moving forward, public health strategies must be grounded in science and equity, free from political interference. The lessons from this pandemic should serve as guiding principles as we strive toward establishing a more resilient and united public health system capable of safeguarding and enhancing the well-being of all individuals. AJPH

CORRESPONDENCE

Correspondence should be sent to Gerardo Chowell, Georgia State University School of Public Health, 140 Decatur St SE, Atlanta, GA 30303 (e-mail: gchowell@gsu.edu). Reprints can be ordered at https://www.ajph.org by clicking the "Reprints" link.

PUBLICATION INFORMATION

Full Citation: Chowell G, Islam N. Political determinants of health: has COVID-19 exposed the worst of it? *Am J Public Health*. 2024;114(9):879–881.

Acceptance Date: June 21, 2024.

DOI: https://doi.org/10.2105/AJPH.2024.307778

ORCID iDs:

Gerardo Chowell https://orcid.org/0000-0003-2194-2251

Nazrul Islam https://orcid.org/0000-0003-3982-4325

CONTRIBUTORS

G. Chowell conceptualized, drafted, and revised the editorial. N. Islam drafted, critically reviewed, and revised the editorial.

CONFLICTS OF INTEREST

The authors report no potential or actual conflicts of interest from funding or affiliation-related activities pertinent to this editorial.

REFERENCES

1. Gadarian SK, Goodman SW, Pepinsky TB. *Pandemic Politics: The Deadly Toll of Partisanship in the Age of COVID*. Princeton, NJ: Princeton University Press; 2022.
2. Gollwitzer A, Martel C, Brady WJ, et al. Partisan differences in physical distancing are linked to health outcomes during the COVID-19 pandemic. *Nat Hum Behav*. 2020;4(11):1186–1197. https://doi.org/10.1038/s41562-020-00977-7
3. Adolph C, Amano K, Bang-Jensen B, et al. Governor partisanship explains the adoption of statewide mask mandates in response to COVID-19. *State Polit Policy Q*. 2022;22(1):24–49. https://doi.org/10.1017/spq.2021.22
4. Kahane LH. Politicizing the mask: political, economic and demographic factors affecting mask wearing behavior in the USA. *East Econ J*. 2021;47(2):163–183. https://doi.org/10.1057/s41302-020-00186-0
5. Kerr J, Panagopoulos C, van der Linden S. Political polarization on COVID-19 pandemic response in the United States. *Pers Individ Dif*. 2021;179:110892. https://doi.org/10.1016/j.paid.2021.110892
6. Ajzenman N, Cavalcanti T, Da Mata D. More than words: leaders' speech and risky behavior during a pandemic. *Am Econ J Econ Policy*. 2023;15(3):351–371. https://doi.org/10.1257/pol.20210284

7. de Almeida L, Carelli PV, Cavalcanti NG, do Nascimento JD, Felinto D. Quantifying political influence on COVID-19 fatality in Brazil. *PLoS One*. 2022;17(7):e0264293. https://doi.org/10.1371/journal.pone.0264293
8. Islam N, Shkolnikov VM, Acosta RJ, et al. Excess deaths associated with COVID-19 pandemic in 2020: age and sex disaggregated time series analysis in 29 high income countries. *BMJ*. 2021;373(1137):n1137. https://doi.org/10.1136/bmj.n1137
9. Nafilyan V, Islam N, Mathur R, et al. Ethnic differences in COVID-19 mortality during the first two waves of the coronavirus pandemic: a nationwide cohort study of 29 million adults in England. *Eur J Epidemiol*. 2021;36(6):605–617. https://doi.org/10.1007/s10654-021-00765-1
10. Islam N, Jdanov DA, Shkolnikov VM, et al. Effects of COVID-19 pandemic on life expectancy and premature mortality in 2020: time series analysis in 37 countries. *BMJ*. 2021;375:e066768. https://doi.org/10.1136/bmj-2021-066768
11. Nafilyan V, Islam N, Ayoubkhani D, et al. Ethnicity, household composition and COVID-19 mortality: a national linked data study. *J R Soc Med*. 2021;114(4):182–211. https://doi.org/10.1177/0141076821999973
12. Benkler Y, Faris R, Roberts H. *Network Propaganda: Manipulation, Disinformation, and Radicalization in American Politics*. New York, NY: Oxford University Press; 2018. https://doi.org/10.1093/oso/9780190923624.001.0001
13. Brownson RC, Chriqui JF, Stamatakis KA. Understanding evidence-based public health policy. *Am J Public Health*. 2009;99(9):1576–1583. https://doi.org/10.2105/AJPH.2008.156224

Excess Death Rates by State During the COVID-19 Pandemic: United States, 2020–2023

Steven H. Woolf, MD, MPH, Jong Hyung Lee, PhD, MS, Derek A. Chapman, PhD, Roy T. Sabo, PhD, and Emily Zimmerman, PhD, MS, MPH

See also Chowell and Islam, p. 879.

Objectives. To estimate state-level excess death rates during 2020 to 2023 and examine differences by region and partisan orientation.

Methods. We modeled death and population counts from the Centers for Disease Control and Prevention to estimate excess death rates for the United States, 9 census divisions, and 50 states. We compared excess death rates for states with different partisan orientations, measured by the party of the seated governor and the level of partisan representation in state legislatures.

Results. The United States experienced 1 277 697 excess deaths between March 2020 and July 2023. Almost 90% of these deaths were attributed to COVID-19, and 51.5% occurred after vaccines were available. The highest excess death rates first occurred in the Northeast and then shifted to the South and Mountain states. Between weeks ending June 20, 2020, through March 19, 2022, excess death rates were higher in states with Republican governors and greater Republican representation in state legislatures.

Conclusions. Excess death rates during the COVID-19 pandemic varied considerably across the US states and were associated with partisan representation in state government, although the influence of confounding variables cannot be excluded. (*Am J Public Health*. 2024;114(9):882–891. https://doi.org/10.2105/AJPH.2024.307731)

AJPH September 2024, Vol. 114, No. 9

The United States experienced a dramatic increase in excess deaths during the COVID-19 pandemic, as many studies have documented.[1–9] "Excess deaths" refers to the difference between observed deaths from all causes and the number that would be expected under normal circumstances. During the COVID-19 pandemic, this difference was largely explained by COVID-19 deaths, but some of the increase reflected deaths attributed to non–COVID-19 causes, such as uncounted or miscoded COVID-19 deaths and deaths among people without COVID-19 who died from other causes induced by the pandemic (e.g., acute emergencies, chronic diseases, behavioral health crises).

The United States experienced more deaths from COVID-19, a higher rate of excess deaths, and larger losses in life expectancy than other high-income countries.[10–13] The US mortality experience was the product of differential mortality trends in the 50 states, but few studies have compared excess death rates at the state level. Previous studies that did report excess death rates by state did so only for 2020 through mid-2021.

Existing state-level data suggest that excess death rates at the onset of the pandemic in spring 2020 were highest in states where the outbreak first occurred (e.g., New York, New Jersey), but patterns shifted over time. As the pandemic spread to other regions, such as the South, states adopted different response plans and experienced disparate mortality outcomes. For example, 1 study found that states that ended lockdowns earlier in May and June of 2020 experienced longer surges in excess deaths during summer 2020 than those that reopened later.[4]

The politicization of public health created a sharp partisan divide in how states responded to the pandemic.[14] In general, states with Republican governors and conservative political orientations were more resistant to enforcement of pandemic control measures (e.g., masking, social distancing, COVID-19 vaccination) than those with Democratic leadership, potentially increasing excess deaths.[15–17] One analysis suggested that more conservative states, notably those in the South, experienced more excess deaths during the Delta-variant surge in fall 2021.[18] Another study reported that excess death rates during June 2020 to April 2022 were higher in states with Republican governors and those with larger Republican representation in the state legislature than states with Democratic governors or a larger Democratic presence in the legislature.[19] A multivariate analysis found that COVID-19 outcomes were not associated with the governor's party but were associated with votes for the 2020 Republican presidential candidate.[20]

In this study, we aimed to estimate state-level excess death rates from 2020 to 2023 and to examine differences by region and partisan orientation. This article contributes to the literature in 4 ways. First, by extending the analysis to 2023, it provides the most current estimates of state-level excess death rates during the COVID-19 pandemic. Second, it compares outcomes across 5 distinct phases of the pandemic, including the initial outbreak, the prevaccine period, and the vaccine period during which vaccination coverage expanded and then stabilized, and a quiescent period during which no major surges in mortality occurred. Third, it compares excess death rates across US Census divisions and states with partisan orientations, measured by both a binary variable (party of the seated governor) and ordinal variable (degree of partisan representation in state legislature). Finally, it employs a sophisticated modeling method to estimate excess deaths and examines the proportion of excess deaths attributed to COVID-19.

METHODS

We obtained weekly death data for the 50 US states and the District of Columbia from the National Center for Health Statistics for the weeks ending March 7, 2020, through the week ending July 1, 2023,[21] and for the same weeks during the preceding 6 years (2014–2019).[22] The analysis included total deaths and deaths from COVID-19. COVID-19 deaths included those in which COVID-19 was cited on death certificates as an underlying or contributing cause. Population counts for 2020 to 2023 were obtained from the projected population counts provided by Centers for Disease Control and Prevention Wide-ranging ONline Data for Epidemiologic Research (CDC WONDER).[23] The partisan orientation of governors and state legislators by year was obtained from the National Conference of State Legislatures.[24] Data on the partisan composition of state legislatures excluded Nebraska, which has a unicameral and nonpartisan legislature.

Estimation of Excess Death Rates

We employed a hierarchical generalized linear mixed model to predict expected deaths based on historical patterns. We estimated expected deaths and their corresponding 95% confidence intervals (CIs) by fitting the model to weekly death counts, assuming a negative binomial distribution to account for potential overdispersion. The analysis covered the period from December 29, 2013, to February 29, 2020, with data drawn from the September 20, 2023, data set.

The selected model, chosen for its optimal fit as detailed in the "Model comparisons" section of the Appendix (available as a supplement to the online version of this article at https://ajph.org), utilized a combination of harmonic functions to account for seasonality and adjusted for annual trends through a continuous year effect. Notably, the model allowed for variations in seasonal and temporal trends at the state level.

We defined excess deaths as the difference between observed and expected deaths predicted by the model. We computed excess death rates by dividing the number of excess deaths by the respective state's population count for the corresponding year.

Phases of Analysis

We calculated the results for the total period (weeks ending March 7, 2020, through July 2, 2023) and for 5 distinct phases of the pandemic:

- Phase 1 (weeks ending March 7, 2020, through June 13, 2020): Phase 1 represents the initial outbreak of the COVID-19 pandemic and the first surge in mortality, which reached its nadir by the week ending June 13, 2020. This phase was marked by lockdowns and increasingly partisan debates over when to reopen and how strongly to trust public health guidance.
- Phase 2 (weeks ending June 20, 2020, through March 13, 2021): Phase 2 represents the prevaccine era, during which state policies on masking, social distancing, and congregate events became more politically polarized. The week ending March 13, 2021, marks the nadir in deaths following the winter 2020–2021 surge.

AJPH September 2024, Vol. 114, No. 9

- Phase 3 (weeks ending March 20, 2021, through March 19, 2022): Phase 3 represents the early vaccine period, during which population uptake of COVID-19 vaccines was increasing and the fall 2021 Delta and Omicron variant surge and the winter 2021–2022 surges occurred. Although COVID-19 vaccines were first available to the public in December 2020, only 24.1% of the US population had received 1 dose as of March 15, 2021, when this phase began.[25] Bollyky et al.[20] marked March 15, 2021, as the start of the vaccine era. This phase ended on March 19, 2022, after completion of the winter 2021–2022 surge and after February 2022, when uptake of COVID-19 vaccines began to plateau, with 76.9% of the population having received 1 dose.[26]
- Phase 4 (weeks ending March 26, 2022, through February 4, 2023): Phase 4 captures the period of stabilizing vaccine coverage and includes the winter 2022–2023 surge, the nation's last major surge in COVID-19 deaths.
- Phase 5 (weeks ending February 11, 2023, through July 2, 2023): Phase 5 captures a relatively quiescent period marked by no major surges.

Analysis by Census Division

In addition to calculating rates at the state level, we also calculated rates for 9 US Census Bureau divisions: Division 1 (New England), Division 2 (Middle Atlantic), Division 3 (East North Central), Division 4 (West North Central), Division 5 (South Atlantic), Division 6 (East South Central), Division 7 (West South Central), Division 8 (Mountain), and Division 9 (Pacific).

Analysis by Partisan Orientation

We stratified excess death rates for each phase based on partisan affiliation, using 3 measures. First, we calculated rates by phase for states with Democratic or Republican governors, based on the party affiliation of the seated governor in the designated year. Second, we calculated rates for states with 4 different levels of Republican representation in the state legislature: less than 33% (group 1), 33% to 49% (group 2), 50% to 66% (group 3), and 67% or more (group 4). Representation of greater than 50% is necessary for party control, and the majority party can exert greater influence if it holds enough seats (usually 67% or greater) to override a governor's veto. Accordingly, the groups were defined to capture Democratic control with (group 1) or without (group 2) veto-override power and Republican control with (group 4) or without (group 3) veto-override power. Third, we calculated rates for states with 4 different levels of control over the branches of government, including 2 "trifecta" scenarios in which either Democrats or Republicans held the governor's seat and controlled both chambers, and 2 scenarios of divided government in which the governor's party controlled only 1 chamber.

Partisan affiliation for each phase was based on data from the National Conference of State Legislatures for the election that immediately preceded the start of each phase. As shown in the Appendix, Tables A through C (available as a supplement to the online version of this article at https://ajph.org), the number of states varied by year for each of the 3 measures (number of governors, by party; level of Republican representation; and control over branches of government). We determined the statistical significance of differences in mortality rates among states grouped by partisan affiliation with the χ^2 test, pairwise comparison of proportions test (with *P* value adjustment utilizing the Benjamini–Hochberg procedure), and the Wilcoxon rank sum test. We conducted data cleaning and preparation in SAS version 9.4 (SAS Institute Inc, Cary, NC), and we conducted statistical analyses in RStudio version 1.3.1093 (RStudio, PBC, Boston, MA).

RESULTS

Over the entire study period (phases 1–5, March 2020 through June 2023), an estimated 1 277 697 excess deaths occurred in the United States, including 1 130 696 (88.5%) deaths attributed to COVID-19. Table 1 provides excess deaths and death rates for the 9 census divisions, the 50 states, and the District of Columbia. Appendix Figures A through E (available as a supplement to the online version of this article at https://ajph.org) map the geographic distribution. Over the course of the entire period, excess death rates were highest in East South Central, Mountain, and West South Central census divisions. The 10 states with the highest excess death rates were West Virginia, New Mexico, Mississippi, South Carolina, Wyoming, Louisiana, Arizona, Kentucky, Arkansas, and Alabama.

Excess Death Rates by Phase

Excess death rates in the United States increased from phase 1 (44.6 per 100 000) to phase 2 (140.7 per 100 000) and phase 3 (150.1 per 100 000) and then fell dramatically during phase 4 (44.6 per 100 000) and phase 5

TABLE 1— Excess Death Rates, by Phase, US Census Divisions, and States: 2020–2023

	Excess Death Rates (per 100 000 Population)					
	Phase 1: Outbreak[a]	Phase 2: Prevaccine[b]	Phase 3: Early Vaccine[c]	Phase 4: Stable Vaccine[d]	Phase 5: Quiescent[e]	Overall[f]
United States	44.6	140.7	150.1	44.6	0.1	94.0
Region 1: Northeast						
Division 1: New England	86.6	46.4	50.1	19.3	−16.3	46.4
Connecticut	119.9	75.5	64.8	26.2	−20.0	66.5
Maine	−1.8	50.6	146.2	80.7	6.8	70.6
Massachusetts	109.6	23.8	17.8	−0.2	−25.0	31.4
New Hampshire	25.1	49.9	72.9	59.7	7.0	53.5
Rhode Island	73.4	86.4	28.5	−31.9	−22.0	33.5
Vermont	17.6	32.6	81.9	47.1	0.8	44.9
Division 2: Mid-Atlantic	149.8	87.7	79.4	4.6	−21.4	74.9
New Jersey	179.5	65.0	46.1	−22.1	−32.6	58.5
New York	200.2	75.0	77.1	25.7	−11.9	91.6
Pennsylvania	50.6	123.9	107.6	−7.9	−27.6	61.6
Region 2: Midwest						
Division 3: East North Central	48.6	130.8	152.8	33.0	−5.3	89.9
Illinois	66.3	115.4	114.4	36.9	−2.3	82.5
Indiana	43.9	152.9	171.7	38.7	−9.6	99.1
Michigan	68.8	97.6	168.1	33.7	−5.8	90.6
Ohio	28.5	171.6	190.6	22.7	−8.6	101.2
Wisconsin	18.2	120.8	115.9	36.5	0.1	72.7
Division 4: West North Central	18.4	137.7	130.5	35.6	−1.4	80.0
Iowa	17.2	137.4	103.7	25.3	−5.7	69.6
Kansas	8.9	164.7	157.6	47.2	8.9	96.7
Minnesota	26.6	76.4	95.8	38.1	4.2	60.0
Missouri	21.5	173.8	180.5	51.9	−1.9	106.1
Nebraska	5.1	111.8	86.8	(2.0)	−3.5	49.5
North Dakota	20.2	200.5	121.6	0.1	−28.7	78.7
South Dakota	0.4	220.7	108.3	(0.9)	−35.2	73.3
Region 3: South						
Division 5: South Atlantic	27.8	144.5	181.8	53.4	0.8	101.0
Delaware	67.1	130.3	168.7	77.7	18.0	115.0
District of Columbia	156.5	151.5	233.2	94.8	17.2	164.7
Florida	13.7	134.7	190.2	37.5	−6.7	90.8
Georgia	31.0	173.5	193.7	56.3	0.7	112.8
Maryland	69.9	100.4	82.6	13.4	−12.8	62.8
North Carolina	17.6	141.0	176.1	63.3	5.8	100.0
South Carolina	28.4	229.4	243.6	80.9	12.8	148.0
Virginia	31.6	116.3	154.9	71.2	12.7	96.1
West Virginia	25.0	195.4	353.2	149.1	17.9	185.5
Division 6: East South Central	25.5	216.5	246.6	59.6	0.9	136.7
Alabama	31.7	243.6	220.1	29.7	−4.0	129.9
Kentucky	18.5	170.5	258.3	86.4	11.6	136.1
Mississippi	50.5	266.9	263.4	78.1	2.7	165.2

Continued

TABLE 1— Continued

	Excess Death Rates (per 100 000 Population)					
	Phase 1: Outbreak[a]	Phase 2: Prevaccine[b]	Phase 3: Early Vaccine[c]	Phase 4: Stable Vaccine[d]	Phase 5: Quiescent[e]	Overall[f]
Tennessee	14.6	204.9	249.8	54.7	−3.3	129.3
Division 7: West South Central	19.1	196.3	185.7	44.5	2.9	111.0
Arkansas	6.0	214.5	228.7	76.4	5.6	132.2
Louisiana	82.6	188.5	225.6	69.5	7.7	143.2
Oklahoma	6.7	207.8	224.3	52.8	−7.2	120.6
Texas	11.6	194.1	169.7	36.1	3.2	102.3
Region 4: West						
Division 8: Mountain	21.7	157.0	193.7	67.9	13.5	112.2
Arizona	26.6	219.3	219.4	87.0	21.8	141.1
Colorado	36.8	98.2	165.4	67.6	16.2	95.5
Idaho	−3.5	97.3	169.7	22.0	−8.9	68.5
Montana	−7.4	138.6	204.2	10.4	−15.1	82.4
Nevada	11.7	160.0	192.1	63.6	12.1	108.1
New Mexico	40.0	220.9	300.1	118.8	31.8	177.7
Utah	5.3	75.8	96.6	25.4	−6.6	48.5
Wyoming	17.4	169.5	262.9	94.0	31.1	143.7
Division 9: Pacific	15.5	135.0	114.2	66.1	16.0	86.1
Alaska	2.2	84.3	225.4	117.4	38.2	116.5
California	18.8	164.3	105.7	61.2	16.1	90.9
Hawaii	−3.2	29.0	95.7	68.1	12.8	50.6
Oregon	4.0	52.2	167.9	94.2	21.2	84.6
Washington	8.2	41.0	123.1	72.4	10.5	63.5

[a]Mar 7, 2020–Jun 13, 2020.
[b]Jun 20, 2020–Mar 13, 2021.
[c]Mar 20, 2021–Mar 19, 2022.
[d]Mar 26, 2022–Feb 4, 2023.
[e]Feb 11, 2023–Jul 2, 2023.
[f]Mar 7, 2020–Jul 2, 2023.

(0.1 per 100 000). Fully 657 945 (51.5%) of the excess deaths (and 580 961 [51.4%] of the deaths attributed to COVID-19) occurred in phases 3 through 5, after COVID-19 vaccines were available. The census divisions and states with the highest excess death rates varied as the pandemic unfolded, with the highest rates first occurring in the Northeast and then shifting to the South and Mountain states.

In phase 1 (March–June 2020), reflecting the outbreak of the pandemic, the Middle Atlantic division experienced the highest excess death rates (149.8 per 100 000), driven by deaths in New York and New Jersey. The 10 states with the nation's highest excess death rates during phase 1 were 2 Middle Atlantic states (New York [200.2 per 100 000], New Jersey [179.5 per 100 000]), 3 New England states (Connecticut [119.9 per 100 000], Massachusetts [109.6 per 100 000], Rhode Island [73.4 per 100 000]), 2 South Atlantic states (Maryland [69.9 per 100 000], Delaware [67.1 per 100 000]), 2 East North Central states (Michigan [68.8 per 100 000], Illinois [66.3 per 100 000]), and 1 West South Central state (Louisiana [82.6 per 100 000]).

In phase 2 (June 2020–March 2021), reflecting the prevaccine era during which excess death rates climbed and pandemic control relied on masking and social distancing, the highest excess death rates occurred in the East South Central, West South Central, and Mountain divisions (216.5 per 100 000, 196.3 per 100 000, and 157.0 per 100 000, respectively). The 10 states with the nation's highest excess death rates during phase 2 were 3 East South

Central states (Mississippi [266.9 per 100 000], Alabama [243.6 per 100 000], Tennessee [204.9 per 100 000]), 2 West South Central states (Arkansas [214.5 per 100 000], Oklahoma [207.8 per 100 000]), 2 Mountain states (New Mexico [220.9 per 100 000], Arizona [219.3 per 100 000]), 2 West North Central states (South Dakota [220.7 per 100 000], North Dakota [200.5 per 100 000]), and 1 South Atlantic state (South Carolina [229.4 per 100 000]).

Phase 3 (March 2021–March 2022) marked the period when COVID-19 vaccines became available—with uptake varying across the country—and when the Delta and Omicron variants caused large surges, producing the nation's highest excess death rates. During this period, the highest excess death rates again occurred in the East South Central, Mountain, and West South Central divisions (246.6 per 100 000, 193.7 per 100 000, and 185.7 per 100 000, respectively). The 10 states with the nation's highest excess death rates were 3 East South Central states (Mississippi [263.4 per 100 000], Kentucky [258.3 per 100 000], Tennessee [249.8 per 100 000]), 2 Mountain states (New Mexico [300.1 per 100 000], Wyoming [262.9 per 100 000]), 2 South Atlantic states (West Virginia [353.2 per 100 000], South Carolina [243.6 per 100 000]), 2 West South Central states (Arkansas [228.7 per 100 000], Louisiana [225.6 per 100 000]), and 1 Pacific state (Alaska [225.4 per 100 000]).

In phase 4 (March 2022–February 2023), during which vaccination uptake stabilized across much of the country and excess death rates declined, the highest excess death rate (67.9 per 100 000) occurred in the Mountain division. The highest excess death rates occurred in 3 Mountain states (New Mexico [118.8 per 100 000], Wyoming [94.0 per 100 000], Arizona [87.0 per 100 000]), 2 South Atlantic states (West Virginia [149.1 per 100 000], South Carolina [80.9 per 100 000]), 2 Pacific states (Alaska [117.4 per 100 000], Oregon [94.2 per 100 000]), 2 East South Central states (Kentucky [86.4 per 100 000], Mississippi [78.1 per 100 000]), and 1 New England state (Maine [80.7 per 100 000]).

In phase 5 (February 2023–July 2023), a period marked by no large surges and negative excess death rates, the Pacific division again experienced the highest rates (16.0 per 100 000). The highest excess death rates occurred in 4 Mountain states (Wyoming [31.1 per 100 000], New Mexico [31.8 per 100 000], Arizona [21.8 per 100 000], Colorado [16.2 per 100 000]), 3 Pacific states (Alaska [38.2 per 100 000], Oregon [21.2 per 100 000], California [16.1 per 100 000]), and 2 South Atlantic states (Delaware [18.0 per 100 000], West Virginia [17.9 per 100 000]).

The lowest excess death rates also varied by phase. By division, the lowest rates occurred in the Pacific and West (North and South) Central divisions in phase 1; New England, Middle Atlantic, and East North Central divisions in phase 2; New England, Middle Atlantic, and Pacific divisions in phase 3; and Middle Atlantic, New England, and East North Central divisions in phase 4. In phase 5, Middle Atlantic, New England, and East and West North Central divisions experienced negative excess death rates.

Excess Death Rates by Partisan Affiliation

States with Republican governors experienced lower excess death rates in phase 1 but significantly higher death rates in phases 2 and 3 than did states with Democratic governors ($P < .001$; Figure 1 and Appendix Table D). In phase 4, excess death rates were slightly higher in states with Democratic governors ($P < .001$). Rates did not differ during phase 5 ($P \geq .99$), the period marked by no COVID-19 surges.

In phases 1 through 3, excess death rates generally exhibited a gradient based on the degree of Republican representation in the state legislature (Figure 2). Increasing Republican representation was associated with lower excess death rates during phase 1 but higher excess death rates during phases 2 and 3 ($P < .001$). States with 33% to 49% of seats occupied by Republicans experienced the lowest death rates in phase 2 and the highest death rates in phase 4 ($P < .001$). No significant differences were observed in phase 5 ($P \geq .99$).

States with unified Republican government (Republican governor and Republican control over both chambers of the legislature) experienced the lowest excess death rates in phase 1 but the highest excess death rates in phases 2 and 3 ($P < .001$; Figure 3). In phase 4, states with unified Democratic government experienced the highest excess death rates ($P < .001$). During phases 2 through 4, states with a Republican governor and a divided legislature had the lowest rates ($P < .001$). No differences were observed in phase 5 ($P \geq .99$).

DISCUSSION

This study estimated that the United States experienced 1 277 697 excess deaths between March 2020 and July 2023, 88.5% of them (1 130 696) involving deaths attributed to COVID-19. More than half (51.4%) of US deaths

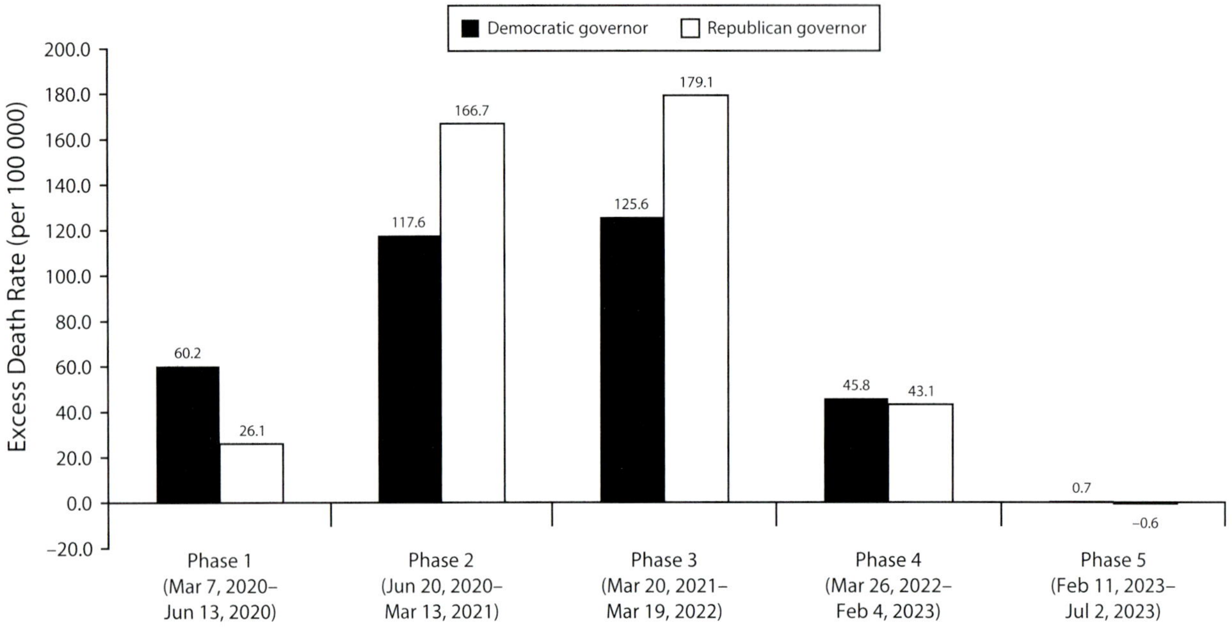

FIGURE 1— Excess Death Rates by Phase and States With Democratic or Republican Governors: United States, 2020–2023

Note. The list of states in each category is provided in Appendix Table A (available as a supplement to the online version of this article at https://doi.org). See Appendix Table D for source data.

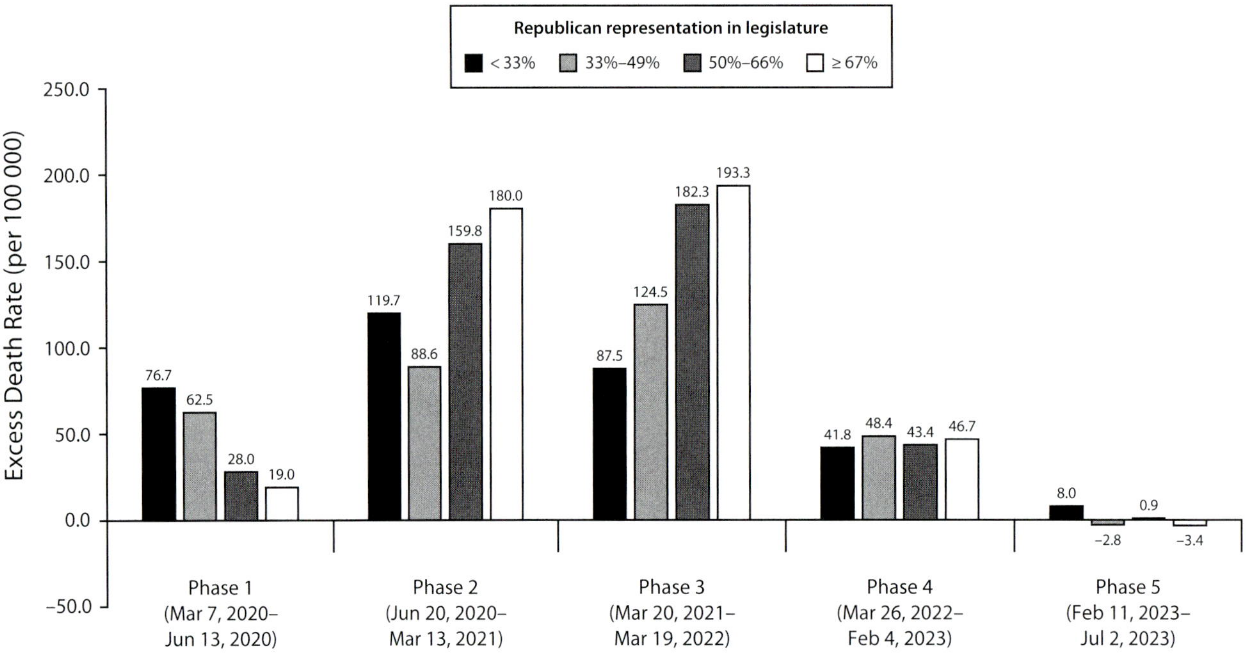

FIGURE 2— Excess Death Rates by Phase and Republican Representation in State Legislature: United States, 2020–2023

Note. The list of states in each category is provided in Appendix Table B (available as a supplement to the online version of this article at https://doi.org). See Appendix Table D for source data.

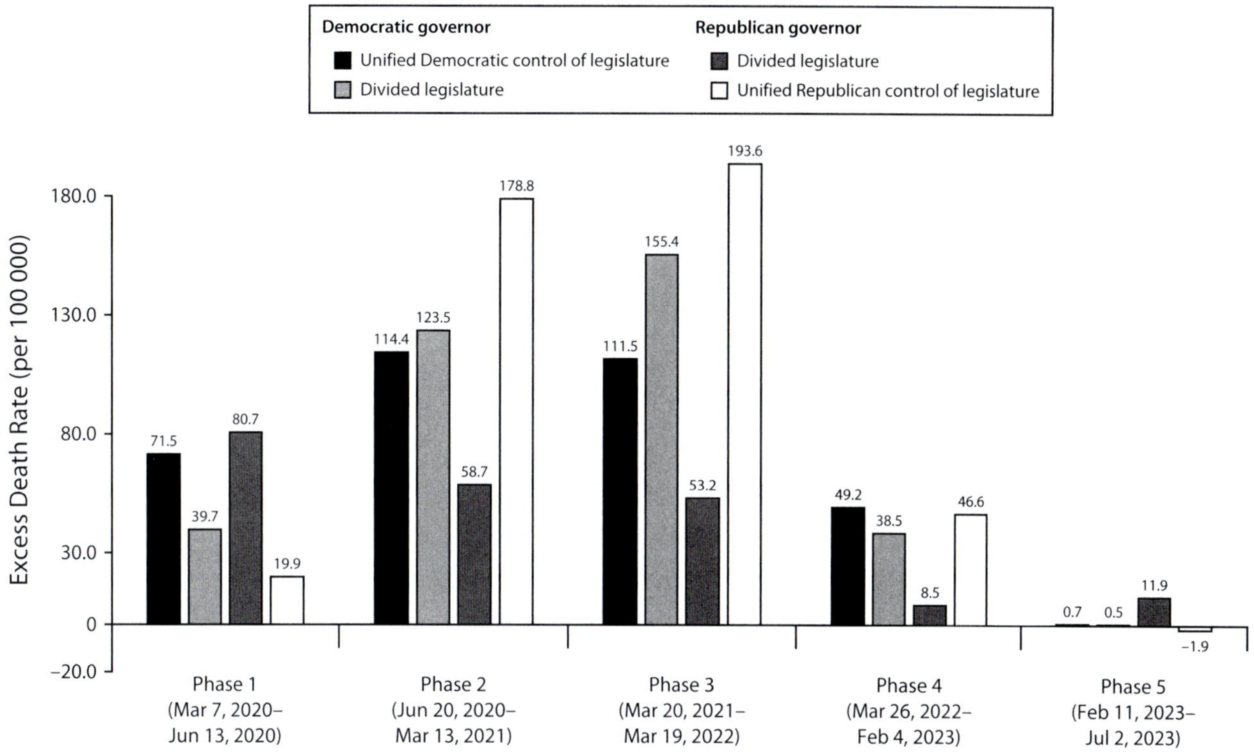

FIGURE 3— **Excess Death Rates by Phase and Partisan Control Over State Government: United States, 2020–2023**

Note. The list of states in each category is provided in Appendix Table C (available as a supplement to the online version of this article at https://ajph.org). See Appendix Table D for source data.

attributed to COVID-19 occurred after COVID-19 vaccines were available (during phases 3 through 5). Observational studies suggest that COVID-19 vaccination could have prevented the majority of these deaths.[26,27] Lower vaccination coverage was predictive of infection and higher mortality rates.[28,29] In addition, many deaths during the prevaccine periods might also have been prevented by greater adherence to masking, social distancing, and other measures to curb viral transmission.

The states with the highest excess death rates varied as the pandemic unfolded. States in the Middle Atlantic census division (e.g., New York, New Jersey) experienced the highest rates at the outbreak of COVID-19, but the high-impact areas then shifted to the South and later to the Mountain states. Understanding the reasons for these geographic patterns will require further research. Some explanations are intuitive: the early concentration in the Middle Atlantic states likely represented the outbreak of the pandemic in large population centers like New York City when this region, like most of the country, did not understand the disease and was unprepared to implement pandemic control measures to prevent rapid transmission of the highly lethal virus.

This study found that states with Republican governors or a larger representation of Republican lawmakers in the legislature generally experienced lower excess death rates in phase 1 (the initial outbreak of COVID-19) and higher rates in phase 2 (the prevaccine period during which pandemic response plans became highly politicized) and phase 3 (the period when the COVID-19 vaccine became available and levels of uptake varied by state). During phases 2 and 3, states with unified Republican control of state government experienced the highest excess death rates, whereas a handful of states with Republican governors and divided legislatures (Maryland, Massachusetts, New Hampshire, and Vermont) experienced the lowest rates. During phase 4—by slight but statistically significant margins—states with Democratic governors and those with unified Democratic control experienced the highest excess death rates.

The association between partisan orientation and excess deaths should be interpreted with caution because the study did not adjust for other potential confounding variables or demonstrate a causal pathway to account for observed outcomes. Potential confounding variables include baseline predisposing characteristics that might have contributed to state variation in excess death rates, such as differences in age distribution, racial/ethnic composition, socioeconomic status, rurality, and the prevalence of comorbid health conditions.[30] For example, calculating age-specific or age-adjusted excess death rates, as others have done, might clarify differences across states for more comparable groups.[1,8] Before the pandemic, counties that voted for Republican presidential candidates experienced higher mortality rates.[31] The populations residing in conservative states often have lower educational attainment, high poverty rates, and diminished access to health care. These and other factors—including a higher prevalence of chronic diseases and other comorbid conditions that increased susceptibility—may have contributed to higher case–fatality rates.

Other sources of confounding include dynamic, time-variant circumstances during the phases of the pandemic, such as viral surges and changes in COVID-19 infection rates, access to health care or personal protective equipment (e.g., masks), and vaccination coverage.[32] Moreover, the populations that predominate in states with certain partisan orientations (and whose voting preferences determine the partisan composition of state government) inhabit different information environments and may have exhibited different attitudes and behaviors that influenced outcomes (e.g., resistance to pandemic control measures, vaccine hesitancy).[33]

Finally, the hypothesis that partisan orientation was associated with excess deaths because of harmful policy choices is compelling but was not formally tested. Doing so would require a complex computing task involving the collection and modeling of thousands of data points to reflect the variety of executive actions, legislation, and court rulings that states enacted, modified, rescinded, and reenacted over time. Examples include stay-in-place orders (lockdowns), masking, restrictions on social distancing and large gatherings, and the implementation and mandating of vaccination.[34] A multivariate analysis that comprehensively accounts for the dynamic change in these policies and adjusts for baseline and dynamic, time-variant confounding variables was beyond the scope of this article but is encouraged for future research. One such analysis suggested that the association between partisan orientation and mortality was attenuated by other covariates.[20]

This study has other limitations that should also be considered. The calculation of excess death rates relied on modeling assumptions and did not account for infection and vaccination rates. Variations in rates across different phases of the pandemic were dependent on the dates chosen for those phases, which likely differed across states and regions. Partisan affiliation was determined based on the most recent election but may have changed during the phase.

Accordingly, the association between partisan orientation and excess death rates is intriguing but must be interpreted with caution, given the potential for interaction effects. The degree to which excess deaths during the COVID-19 pandemic reflect policy choices by elected officials warrants further research using study designs that can isolate the independent effects of policy contexts. AJPH

ABOUT THE AUTHORS

Steven H. Woolf and Jong Hyung Lee are with the Department of Family Medicine, Virginia Commonwealth University (VCU) School of Medicine, Richmond. Derek A. Chapman and Emily Zimmerman are with the Department of Epidemiology, VCU School of Population Health, Richmond. Roy T. Sabo is with the Department of Biostatistics, VCU School of Population Health.

CORRESPONDENCE

Correspondence should be sent to Steven H. Woolf, MD, MPH, Center on Society and Health, Virginia Commonwealth University School of Medicine, 830 E Main St, Suite 5035, Richmond, VA 23298-0212 (e-mail: steven.woolf@vcuhealth.org). Reprints can be ordered at https://www.ajph.org by clicking the "Reprints" link.

PUBLICATION INFORMATION

Full Citation: Woolf SH, Lee JH, Chapman DA, Sabo RT, Zimmerman E. Excess death rates by state during the COVID-19 pandemic: United States, 2020–2023. *Am J Public Health*. 2024;114(9):882–891.

Acceptance Date: May 17, 2024.

DOI: https://doi.org/10.2105/AJPH.2024.307731

ORCID iDs:
Steven H. Woolf https://orcid.org/0000-0001-9384-033X

Derek A. Chapman https://orcid.org/0000-0001-5872-8561

Roy T. Sabo https://orcid.org/0000-0001-9159-4876

Emily Zimmerman https://orcid.org/0000-0003-2678-6657

CONTRIBUTORS

S. H. Woolf was responsible for conceptualizing the study, interpreting the data, and writing the article. J. H. Lee and D. A. Chapman were responsible for data modeling and calculation of excess death rates, with biostatistical guidance provided by R. T. Sabo. J. H. Lee, D. A. Chapman, R. T. Sabo, and E. Zimmerman provided input on study design and helped edit the article. J. H. Lee produced the maps.

ACKNOWLEDGMENTS

S. H. Woolf received partial funding from the National Center for Advancing Translational Sciences (grant UM1TR004360).

CONFLICTS OF INTEREST

The authors have no conflicts of interest to report.

HUMAN PARTICIPANT PROTECTION

Informed consent for the study was not required because human participants were not involved.

REFERENCES

1. Rossen LM, Branum AM, Ahmad FB, Sutton P, Anderson RN. Excess deaths associated with COVID-19, by age and race and ethnicity—United

States, January 26–October 3, 2020. *MMWR Morb Mortal Wkly Rep*. 2020;69(42):1522–1527. https://doi.org/10.15585/mmwr.mm6942e2

2. Weinberger DM, Chen J, Cohen T, et al. Estimation of excess deaths associated with the COVID-19 pandemic in the United States, March to May 2020. *JAMA Intern Med*. 2020;180(10):1336–1344. https://doi.org/10.1001/jamainternmed.2020.3391
3. Rossen LM, Ahmad FB, Anderson RN, et al. Disparities in excess mortality associated with COVID-19—United States, 2020. *MMWR Morb Mortal Wkly Rep*. 2021;70(33):1114–1119. https://doi.org/10.15585/mmwr.mm7033a2
4. Woolf SH, Chapman DA, Sabo RT, Weinberger DM, Hill L, Taylor DDH. Excess deaths from COVID-19 and other causes, March–July 2020. *JAMA*. 2020;324(15):1562–1564. https://doi.org/10.1001/jama.2020.19545
5. Cronin CJ, Evans WN. Excess mortality from COVID and non-COVID causes in minority populations. *Proc Natl Acad Sci U S A*. 2021;118(39):e2101386118. https://doi.org/10.1073/pnas.2101386118
6. Shiels MS, Haque AT, Haozous EA, et al. Racial and ethnic disparities in excess deaths during the COVID-19 pandemic, March to December 2020. *Ann Intern Med*. 2021;174(12):1693–1699. https://doi.org/10.7326/M21-2134
7. Ruhm CJ. Excess deaths in the United States during the first year of COVID-19. *Prev Med*. 2022;162:107174. https://doi.org/10.1016/j.ypmed.2022.107174
8. Ludden IG, Jacobson SH, Jokela JA. Excess deaths by sex and age group in the first two years of the COVID-19 pandemic in the United States. *Health Care Manag Sci*. 2022;25(3):515–520. https://doi.org/10.1007/s10729-022-09606-3
9. Rossen LM, Nørgaard SK, Sutton PD, et al. Excess all-cause mortality in the USA and Europe during the COVID-19 pandemic, 2020 and 2021. *Sci Rep*. 2022;12(1):18559. https://doi.org/10.1038/s41598-022-21844-7
10. Islam N, Shkolnikov VM, Acosta RJ, et al. Excess deaths associated with COVID-19 pandemic in 2020: age and sex disaggregated time series analysis in 29 high income countries. *BMJ*. 2021;373(1137):n1137. https://doi.org/10.1136/bmj.n1137
11. COVID-19 Excess Mortality Collaborators. Estimating excess mortality due to the COVID-19 pandemic: a systematic analysis of COVID-19-related mortality, 2020–21. *Lancet*. 2022;399(10334):1513–1536. https://doi.org/10.1016/S0140-6736(21)02796-3
12. Bilinski A, Thompson K, Emanuel E. COVID-19 and excess all-cause mortality in the US and 20 comparison countries, June 2021–March 2022. *JAMA*. 2023;329(1):92–94. https://doi.org/10.1001/jama.2022.21795
13. Msemburi W, Karlinsky A, Knutson V, Aleshin-Guendel S, Chatterji S, Wakefield J. The WHO estimates of excess mortality associated with the COVID-19 pandemic. *Nature*. 2023;613(7942):130–137. https://doi.org/10.1038/s41586-022-05522-2
14. Adolph C, Amano K, Bang-Jensen B, Fullman N, Wilkerson J. Pandemic politics: timing state-level social distancing responses to COVID-19. *J Health Polit Policy Law*. 2021;46(2):211–233. https://doi.org/10.1215/03616878-8802162
15. Goldmacher S. GOP governors fight mandates as the party's Covid politics harden. *New York Times*. August 31, 2021. Available at: https://www.nytimes.com/2021/08/31/us/politics/republican-governors-covid-19.html. Accessed May 4, 2022.
16. Hubler S, Cowan J. Flurry of new laws move blue and red states further apart. *New York Times*. April 3, 2022. Available at: https://www.nytimes.com/2022/04/03/us/state-laws-republican-democrat-division.html. Accessed May 4, 2022.
17. Warner ME, Zhang X. Social safety nets and COVID-19 stay home orders across US states: a comparative policy analysis. *J Comp Policy Anal*. 2021;23(2):176–190. https://doi.org/10.1080/13876988.2021.1874243
18. Woolf SH. The growing influence of state governments on population health in the United States. *JAMA*. 2022;327(14):1331–1332. https://doi.org/10.1001/jama.2022.3785
19. Woolf SH, Sabo RT, Chapman DA, Lee JH. Association between partisan affiliation of state governments and state mortality rates before and during the COVID-19 pandemic. *Milbank Q*. 2023;101(4):1191–1222; https://doi.org/10.1111/1468-0009.12672
20. Bollyky TJ, Castro E, Aravkin AY, et al. Assessing COVID-19 pandemic policies and behaviours and their economic and educational trade-offs across US states from Jan 1, 2020, to July 31, 2022: an observational analysis. *Lancet*. 2023;401(10385):1341–1360. https://doi.org/10.1016/S0140-6736(23)00461-0
21. Centers for Disease Control and Prevention. Weekly counts of deaths by state and select causes, 2020–2023. Available at: https://data.cdc.gov/NCHS/Weekly-Counts-of-Deaths-by-State-and-Select-Causes/muzy-jte6. Accessed September 20, 2023.
22. Centers for Disease Control and Prevention. Weekly counts of deaths by state and select causes, 2014–2019. Available at: https://data.cdc.gov/NCHS/Weekly-Counts-of-Deaths-by-State-and-Select-Causes/3yf8-kanr. Accessed August 18, 2023.
23. CDC WONDER. Population projections. United States, 2004–2030, by state, age, and sex. Available at: http://wonder.cdc.gov/population-projections.html. Accessed August 4, 2023.
24. National Conference of State Legislatures. State partisan composition. Available at: https://www.ncsl.org/about-state-legislatures/state-partisan-composition. Accessed September 22, 2023.
25. Centers for Disease Control and Prevention. COVID-19 vaccination trends in the United States, national and jurisdictional. Available at: https://data.cdc.gov/Vaccinations/COVID-19-Vaccination-Trends-in-the-United-States-N/rh2h-3yt2. Accessed November 10, 2023.
26. Tenforde MW, Self WH, Gaglani M, et al. IVY Network. Effectiveness of mRNA vaccination in preventing COVID-19–associated invasive mechanical ventilation and death—United States, March 2021–January 2022. *MMWR Morb Mortal Wkly Rep*. 2022;71(12):459–465. https://doi.org/10.15585/mmwr.mm7112e1
27. DeCuir J, Surie D, Zhu Y, et al. Effectiveness of monovalent mRNA COVID-19 vaccination in preventing COVID-19–associated invasive mechanical ventilation and death among immunocompetent adults during the Omicron variant period—IVY Network, 19 US States, February 1, 2022–January 31, 2023. *MMWR Morb Mortal Wkly Rep*. 2023;72:463–468. https://doi.org/10.15585/mmwr.mm7217a3
28. Cuadros DF, Miller FD, Awad S, Coule P, MacKinnon NJ. Analysis of vaccination rates and new COVID-19 infections by US county, July–August 2021. *JAMA Netw Open*. 2022;5(2):e2147915. https://doi.org/10.1001/jamanetworkopen.2021.47915
29. Cuadros DF, Moreno CM, Musuka G, Miller FD, Coule P, MacKinnon NJ. Association between vaccination coverage disparity and the dynamics of the COVID-19 Delta and Omicron waves in the US. *Front Med (Lausanne)*. 2022;9:898101. https://doi.org/10.3389/fmed.2022.898101
30. Kelly G, Petti S, Noah N. Covid-19, non-Covid-19 and excess mortality rates not comparable across countries. *Epidemiol Infect*. 2021;149:e176. https://doi.org/10.1017/S0950268821001850
31. Warraich HJ, Kumar P, Nasir K, Joynt Maddox KE, Wadhera RK. Political environment and mortality rates in the United States, 2001–19: population based cross sectional analysis. *BMJ*. 2022;377:e069308. https://doi.org/10.1136/bmj-2021-069308
32. Pallari CT, Achilleos S, Quattrocchi A. Magnitude and determinants of excess total, age-specific and sex-specific all-cause mortality in 24 countries worldwide during 2020 and 2021: results on the impact of the COVID-19 pandemic from the C-MOR project. *BMJ Glob Health*. 2024;9(4):e013018. https://doi.org/10.1136/bmjgh-2023-013018
33. Dowd-Arrow B, Burdette AM, Smith A. Political variations in pandemic lifestyles and COVID-19 vaccination by age cohort in the United States. *Prev Med*. 2023;172:107525. https://doi.org/10.1016/j.ypmed.2023.107525
34. Hill T, Gonzalez K, Davis A. The nastiest question: does population mobility vary by state political ideology during the novel coronavirus (COVID-19) pandemic? *Sociol Perspect*. 2021;64(5):786–803. https://doi.org/10.1177/0731121420979700

Psychosocial Syndemic Burden, Sexual Behaviors, and Engagement in HIV Prevention Care Among Sexual and Gender Minority Youths: United States, 2022

Pablo K. Valente, MD, PhD, MPH, Raghavee Neupane, MPH, Lisa Eaton, PhD, and Ryan J. Watson, PhD

Objectives. To examine linear and nonlinear associations between psychosocial syndemic factors and HIV risk and engagement in HIV prevention care among sexual and gender minority (SGM) youths.

Methods. Between February and October 2022, we recruited 17 578 SGM youths aged 13 to 18 years in the United States for an online survey. We examined the relationship of syndemics (i.e., binge drinking, drug use, sexual victimization, and anti–lesbian, gay, bisexual, and transgender discrimination) with sexual behaviors (i.e., sexual initiation, condomless anal or vaginal sex, and number of sexual partners) and HIV prevention care (i.e., HIV testing, preexposure prophylaxis awareness and utilization) using regression.

Results. Psychosocial syndemic burden (number of syndemic factors reported) was linearly and cubically associated with engagement in sexual behaviors. Psychosocial syndemic burden was linearly associated with higher HIV testing and preexposure prophylaxis awareness and cubically associated with higher preexposure prophylaxis utilization.

Conclusions. Our findings are evidence of synergism across psychosocial syndemic factors regarding HIV risk and engagement in HIV prevention care among SGM youths in the United States.

Public Health Implications. Multicomponent interventions may help reduce HIV risk and promote access to HIV prevention services among SGM individuals aged 13 to 18 years. (*Am J Public Health*. 2024;114(9):892–902. https://doi.org/10.2105/AJPH.2024.307753)

AJPH September 2024, Vol. 114, No. 9

Sexual and gender minority (SGM) youths aged 13 to 24 years bear a disproportionate burden of the HIV epidemic, accounting for more than 80% of new HIV diagnoses in their age group.[1] Behaviors associated with HIV transmission, including condomless sex, multiple sexual partners, and sexualized drug use, are more prevalent among SGM youths than among their heterosexual counterparts, contributing to heightened HIV risk among this population.[2,3] Suboptimal engagement in HIV prevention care among SGM youths also contributes to continued HIV transmission.[4] In particular, preexposure prophylaxis (PrEP) uptake among youths younger than 18 years is low, with only 1.1% of commercially insured individuals in the United States with PrEP indications having received a prescription.[5]

Increased HIV risk and lower engagement in care cooccur with psychosocial problems, commonly referred to as syndemics. Initially developed to explain interrelationships between substance use, violence, and HIV risk,[6] the concept of syndemics has been expanded to include factors such as depression,[7,8] alcohol use,[8,9] stigma,[10] and poverty.[7] There is robust evidence that several syndemic factors are more prevalent among SGM youths than among their heterosexual counterparts.[3,11–13] Mounting evidence also shows that syndemic factors are associated with behaviors that may lead to HIV acquisition (e.g., condomless sex),[9,14] increased HIV and sexually transmitted infection transmission,[8] and poor engagement in HIV treatment and prevention care[15,16] among SGM youths and adults.

Much of the literature on syndemics has focused on demonstrating additive dose–response relationships between syndemic factors and negative health and social outcomes.[7,8,10,14] These studies show linear, progressive worsening of social and health conditions as the number of syndemic factors experienced increases. However, these studies are not able to adequately examine whether syndemic factors interact with one another to contribute to negative health outcomes, a key assumption of syndemic theory.[17,18] The distinction between additive and synergistic relationships is of relevance because the latter would suggest that interventions addressing more than 1 syndemic factor would likely have greater health and social effects.[19]

Studies examining syndemic interactions have found conflicting results. For example, Tomori et al. found a significant dose–response relationship between the number of syndemic conditions and condomless anal sex and a similar, albeit not statistically significant, pattern for syphilis.[20] Synergistic interactions were observed between intimate partner violence and depression for condomless anal sex, and between alcohol dependence and illicit drug use for syphilis.[20] Similarly, Bulled identified synergism between substance use and violence with respect to HIV infection among White individuals but not individuals of color.[21] Other studies examining interactions between syndemic factors have found inconsistent results, including null findings[22] or antagonistic interactions (the combined effect of 2 syndemic factors being smaller than the sum of the individual effects of each).[23]

Inconsistent findings regarding synergism across studies (i.e., different pairs of syndemic factors showing significant interaction) and within studies (i.e., different interaction results for similar outcomes, such as condomless sex and sexually transmitted infections[20]) make interpretation of findings and their implications less clear. Additionally, research that focused on 2-way interactions may fail to capture more complex interrelationships across multiple syndemic factors, which is at the core of theoretical conceptualizations of syndemics.[18] Moreover, although several studies have examined relationships between psychosocial syndemics and HIV-related outcomes among SGM youths, few studies have focused on individuals younger than 18 years. The transition from adolescence to young adulthood is marked by changes in how SGM individuals experience psychosocial problems and HIV risk,[12,24] and engagement in HIV prevention care is especially low among individuals younger than 18 years.[5] Therefore, the dearth of studies with SGM individuals younger than 18 years is another important gap in the existing literature.

To address these gaps, we examined linear and synergistic associations between psychosocial syndemic burden (i.e., an index that included substance use, binge drinking, sexual victimization, and anti-LGBTQ [lesbian, gay, bisexual, transgender, queer or questioning] discrimination) and HIV risk and engagement in HIV preventive care in a large online US sample of SGM youths aged 13 to 18 years.

METHODS

Between February and October 2022, we recruited SGM youths online through social media ads, collaborations with social media influencers aligned with the LGBTQ community, and community- and school-based organizations.[25] Individuals were eligible to participate if they were aged 13 to 18 years; identified as a sexual minority (e.g., lesbian, gay, bisexual, pansexual), gender minority (e.g., transgender, nonbinary, agender), or both; and lived in the United States.

Individuals took a screener survey and, if eligible, received a link to the online survey. To identify duplicate and fraudulent responses, research staff examined e-mail and IP (Internet protocol) addresses, attention-check questions, time to complete survey, response patterns, and write-in questions for unusual or suspicious patterns. Additionally, we asked individuals without institutional e-mail accounts to verify their identities with pictures of their IDs or video calls with research staff to receive remuneration. Of 24 570 individuals who we found eligible and who consented or assented to study participation, we excluded 6992 who were deemed fraudulent or duplicate or had less than 9% survey completion (i.e., completed demographic questions). This resulted in 17 578 individuals with demographic data, of which we had complete data for 9480 individuals (~54%). The most common missing data pattern was abandoning the survey immediately after demographic questions.

Measures

HIV risk behaviors. We assessed the following factors associated with HIV transmission: sexual initiation, defined as previous vaginal, anal, or oral sexual activity (yes/no); condomless anal or vaginal sex (CAVS) in the past 3 months (yes/no); and number of sexual partners in the past 3 months (winsorized at 6 partners).

Engagement in HIV prevention care. We assessed PrEP awareness ("Have you heard of PrEP?", yes/no) and PrEP utilization ("Have you ever taken PrEP in your life?", yes/no) among all participants. We also asked individuals who reported sexual initiation about whether they had ever been tested for HIV (yes/no).

Psychosocial syndemic burden. Similar to previous studies,[10,14] we created a count score of psychosocial syndemic burden ranging from 0 to 4, with higher scores indicating higher exposure to syndemics. We considered 4 syndemic indicators:

1. Recent binge drinking. We assessed the number of times participants had 5 or more drinks of alcohol within a couple of hours in the past 30 days. We dichotomized responses as any versus no recent binge drinking.
2. Lifetime drug use. We asked participants whether they had ever used drugs not prescribed by a doctor, such as stimulants, opioids, and hallucinogens, but excluding alcohol, nicotine, and cannabis. We dichotomized responses as any versus no drug use.
3. Sexual victimization and rape. With the following question, we assessed whether participants had been sexually victimized or raped: "Have you ever been physically forced to have sexual intercourse when you did not want to?" We dichotomized responses as yes versus no.
4. Anti-LGBTQ discrimination. We assessed how often participants had been teased, threatened, or harassed about being LGBTQ in the past 12 months (ranging from "never" to "very often"). We assessed in-person and online discrimination separately and then combined responses into a single dichotomous anti-LGBTQ discrimination measure (any vs no anti-LGBTQ discrimination).

Depressive symptoms. We assessed symptoms of depressive mood in the past 2 weeks with the Patient Health Questionnaire-2, a 2-item screening tool for major depression.[26] Responses to both questions ranged from 0 ("not at all") to 3 ("nearly every day"). We summed responses and considered them to potentially indicate major depression for scores of 3 or higher, as previously recommended.[26]

We also assessed age, race/ethnicity, sex assigned at birth, sexual orientation, and gender identity.

Analysis

To examine the cooccurrence of psychosocial problems, we examined pairwise associations between hypothesized syndemic factors using logistic regression. We then examined relationships between psychosocial syndemics and depressive symptoms (independent variables) and HIV risk and engagement in HIV prevention care (dependent variables) using linear and logistic regression for continuous and categorical outcomes, respectively. Because depressive symptoms diverged from other syndemic factors in their associations with our outcomes, we included depressive symptoms separately in our models.[17]

We explored syndemic synergism with the inclusion of psychosocial syndemic burden as a categorical variable in saturated regression models. We also explored *P* values for linear, quadratic, and cubic trends and obtained adjusted predicted means (for continuous outcomes) and probabilities (for binary outcomes) considering the highest-order significant ($P < .05$) polynomial term for the effect of psychosocial syndemic burden. Adjusted analyses controlled for age, race/ethnicity, sexual orientation, gender identity, sex assigned at birth, and highest level of education of parents or caregivers. We also conducted post hoc analyses for PrEP outcomes adjusting for HIV risk behaviors to assess the potential mediating role of sexual behaviors, and we examined potential interaction by race/ethnicity and gender identity.

To account for missing data, we conducted sensitivity analyses using 50 imputed data sets, using chained equations and predictive mean matching for continuous variables and logit regression for categorical ones.

We conducted data analyses in Stata/SE version 17.0 (StataCorp LP, College Station, TX).

RESULTS

Participants in our study had a mean age of 15.79 years (SD = 1.49 years). Most were assigned female sex at birth (61.8%) and identified as White (69.9%), with 18.2% reporting Latinx ethnicity. Our sample was diverse in sexual orientation (29.3% identified as gay or lesbian, 28.5% as bisexual, and 14.6% as pansexual) and gender identity (19.3% identified as a cisgender boy, 16.7% as a transgender boy, 16.2% as a cisgender girl, and 15.2% as nonbinary). There were participants from all 50 US states, with 33% from the US South, 24.2% from the West, 23.3% from the Midwest, and 19.5% from the Northeast. Supplemental Table A (available as a supplement to the online version of this article at http://www.ajph.org) shows the sociodemographic characteristics of our sample. Individuals with incomplete data were more likely to be younger, assigned male at birth, non-White, straight identified, and cisgender (all $P < .001$, not shown).

Psychosocial Syndemics and Depressive Symptoms

Psychosocial syndemic factors were commonly reported among our sample. About three quarters reported at least 1 psychosocial syndemic factor (n = 7700; 73.8%), such as anti-LGBTQ discrimination (n = 7908; 69.8%), sexual victimization or rape (n = 1509; 14.4%), recent binge drinking (n = 737; 6.7%), and lifetime drug use (n = 695; 6.3%). About one half of the sample screened positive for depression (n = 5882; 55.0%; Supplemental Table A).

All hypothesized syndemic factors, including depressive symptoms, were positively associated with one another (all $P < .001$), indicating cooccurrence of syndemic indicators. Supplemental Table B (available as a supplement to the online version of this article at http://www.ajph.org) shows bivariate associations between hypothesized syndemic factors.

Psychosocial Syndemics and Sexual Behaviors

About one fourth of the sample reported sexual activity ever (n = 2984; 27.5%), and 84% reported no sexual partners in the past 3 months (average number of partners in the period was 0.23; SD = 0.68). CAVS in the past 3 months was reported by 8.3% of the sample (n = 870; Supplemental Table A).

Psychosocial syndemic burden was additively associated with sexual behaviors (Table 1). Sexual initiation was progressively more common as the number of syndemic factors increased: coefficients ranged from adjusted odds ratio (AOR) = 1.70 (95% confidence interval [CI] = 1.49, 1.94) among individuals with 1 syndemic factor to AOR = 84.28 (95% CI = 35.65, 199.24) for those with all 4 syndemic factors, compared with individuals reporting no syndemic factors ($P < .001$ for linear trend; $P = .49$ for quadratic trend; $P = .07$ for cubic trend). Depressive symptoms were not associated with sexual initiation (AOR = 0.96; 95% CI = 0.90, 1.33).

Similarly, CAVS was progressively more common for individuals with a higher syndemic burden (AOR = 1.78; 95% CI = 1.40, 2.26 for 1 syndemic factor and AOR = 31.81; 95% CI = 18.86, 53.66 for 4 syndemic factors; $P < .001$ for linear trend, $P = .96$ for quadratic trend, and $P = .04$ for cubic trend). Depressive symptoms were not associated with CAVS (AOR = 0.90; 95% CI = 0.76, 1.06). Number of sexual partners was also cumulatively associated with syndemics (b = 0.08; 95% CI = 0.06, 0.11 for 1 syndemic factor, and b = 1.69; 95% CI = 1.56, 1.83 for 4 syndemic factors; with $P < .001$ for linear trend, $P < .001$ for quadratic trend, and $P = .01$ for cubic trend). Depressive symptoms were not associated with the number of sexual partners (b = −0.02; 95% CI = −0.04, 0.01).

Predicted probabilities and means shown in Figure 1 indicate nonlinear relationships between the psychosocial syndemic burden and sexual behavior outcomes. Specifically, there is multiplicative growth in the probability of CAVS as the number of syndemic factors increase (Figure 1b), with growth leveling off toward higher numbers of syndemic factors. Regarding the number of sexual partners, multiplicative growth does not appear to plateau in the observed range of syndemic exposure (Figure 1c).

Psychosocial Syndemics and HIV Prevention Care

Utilization of HIV prevention care was low among our sample. Among individuals who reported sexual initiation, 15.8% (n = 471) had been tested for HIV. In the overall sample, 26.2% (n = 2844) were aware of PrEP for HIV prevention and only 1.1% had ever utilized PrEP (n = 114).

Contrary to expectations, syndemic burden was positively associated with engagement in HIV care (Table 2). Among participants reporting sexual initiation, HIV testing was progressively more common among individuals with higher syndemic burden: AOR = 1.42 (95% CI = 0.97, 2.09) among individuals with 1 syndemic factor, and AOR = 7.25 (95% CI = 3.97, 13.25; $P < .001$ for linear trend, $P = .75$ for quadratic trend, and $P = .41$ for cubic trend). Depressive symptoms were not associated with HIV testing (AOR = 0.88; 95% CI = 0.69, 1.11).

Syndemic burden was also progressively associated with PrEP awareness (ranging from AOR = 1.12; 95% CI = 1.00, 1.26 for 1 syndemic factor to AOR = 2.43; 95% CI = 1.53, 3.86 for 4 factors; $P < .001$ for linear trend, $P = .36$ for quadratic trend, $P = .30$ for cubic trend). Depressive symptoms were

TABLE 1— Associations Between Psychosocial Syndemic Burden and Sexual Behaviors: United States, February–October 2022

	Sexual Initiation (n = 9888 in Adjusted Models)			CAVS (3 Mo) (n = 9496 in Adjusted Models)			Number of Sexual Partners (3 Mo) (n = 9887 in Adjusted Models)		
	$n_{(event)}$ Yes/No[a]	AOR (95% CI)[b]	P for Trend	$n_{(event)}$ Yes/No[a]	AOR (95% CI)[b]	P for trend	Mean ±SD[c]	AOR[b] (95% CI)[b]	P for trend
Psychosocial syndemic burden, no. of syndemic factors			Linear: < .001; Quadratic: .49; Cubic: .07			Linear: < .001; Quadratic: .97; Cubic: .04			Linear: < .001; Quadratic: < .001; Cubic: .01
0	431/2296	1 (Ref)		110/2549	1 (Ref)		0.11 ±0.41	1 (Ref)	
1	1217/4561	1.70 (1.49, 1.94)		314/5251	1.78 (1.40, 2.26)		0.16 ±0.52	0.08 (0.06, 0.11)	
2	873/628	9.40 (7.98, 11.08)		251/1149	6.21 (4.79, 8.05)		0.46 ±0.91	0.36 (0.32, 0.41)	
3	256/66	25.35 (18.53, 34.68)		106/193	15.07 (10.81, 21.02)		0.92 ±1.29	0.80 (0.73, 0.87)	
4	82/7	84.28 (35.65, 199.24)		48/38	31.81 (18.86, 53.66)		1.79 ±1.90	1.69 (1.56, 1.83)	
Depressive symptoms									
Yes	1620/4103	0.96 (0.90, 1.33)		463/5033	0.90 (0.76, 1.06)		0.22 ±0.65	−0.02 (−0.04, 0.01)	
No	1205/3462	1 (Ref)		349/4134	1 (Ref)		0.23 ±0.66	1 (Ref)	

Note. AOR = adjusted odds ratio; CAVS = condomless anal or vaginal sex; CI = confidence interval. Regression models considered psychosocial syndemic burden as a categorical variable and assessed linear, quadratic, and cubic trends.
[a]Number of individuals reporting the outcome of interest (i.e., sexual initiation, CAVS) and not reporting the outcome of interest by level of the covariate.
[b]Adjusted models controlled for the effects of age, race/ethnicity, gender identity, sex assigned at birth, and sexual orientation.
[c]Mean ±SD of outcome of interest (number of sexual partners) by level of the covariate.

negatively associated with PrEP awareness (AOR = 0.82; 95% CI = 0.74, 0.90). Finally, there was also a cumulative association between syndemic burden and lifetime PrEP utilization, ranging from AOR = 1.42 (95% CI = 0.67, 2.97) for 1 syndemic factor to AOR = 35.73 (95% CI = 13.40, 95.28) for 4 syndemic factors ($P < .001$ for linear trend, $P = .98$ for quadratic trend, and $P = .01$ for cubic trend). Depressive symptoms were not associated with PrEP utilization (AOR = 0.85; 95% CI = 0.55, 1.302).

As shown in Figure 2a and 2b, the probabilities of previous HIV testing and PrEP awareness increased linearly with the psychosocial syndemic burden. Figure 2c shows multiplicative growth in the probability of PrEP utilization by syndemic burden and an indication of a potential plateau in the upper range of observed psychosocial syndemic burden, although with wide CIs.

Post Hoc Analyses

To probe the unexpected association between psychosocial syndemic burden and greater, rather than lower, engagement in PrEP care, we conducted further analyses controlling for the effect of sexual behaviors that could be proxies for PrEP indication (i.e., sexual initiation, CAVS, and number of sexual partners). These models indicated that the relationship between psychosocial syndemic burden and previous HIV testing, PrEP awareness, and PrEP utilization remained positive, yet with a smaller magnitude (Table 2). Additionally, the number of sexual partners was associated with PrEP awareness (AOR = 1.14; 95% CI = 1.04, 1.25) and PrEP utilization (AOR = 1.28; 95% CI = 1.07, 1.53). Sexual initiation was associated with PrEP awareness only (AOR = 1.25; 95% CI = 1.09, 1.44), and

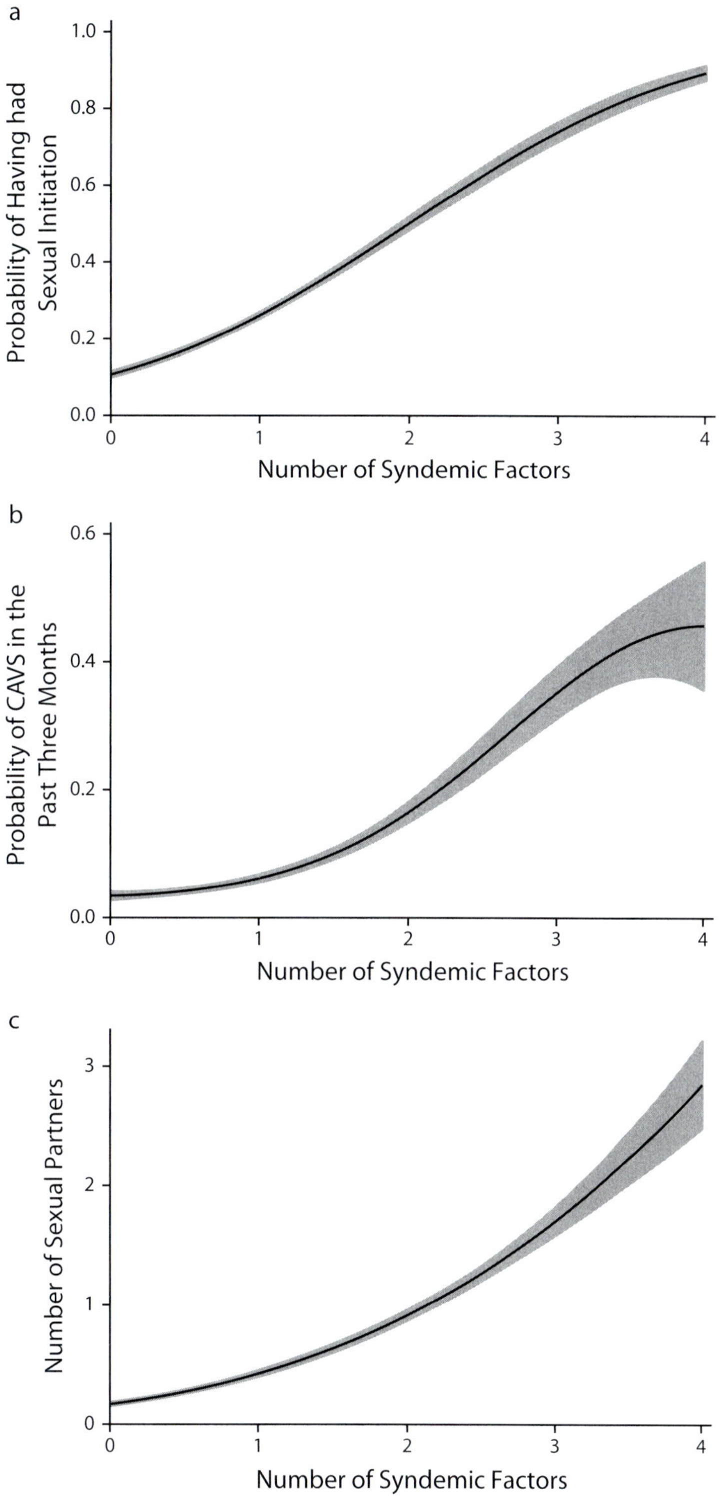

FIGURE 1— **Number of Reported Psychosocial Syndemic Factors Based on Highest-Order Significant Polynomial Regression Model and Adjusted Predicted Probabilities and Means of (a) Sexual Initiation, (b) Condomless Anal or Vaginal Sex (CAVS), and (c) Number of Sexual Partners: United States, February–October 2022**

Note. Part a shows linear models, and parts b and c show cubic models of the predicted probabilities of sexual behavior outcomes and psychosocial syndemic burden. In all models, psychosocial syndemic burden was considered as a continuous predictor. Adjusted models controlled for the effects of age, race/ethnicity, gender identity, sex assigned at birth, and sexual orientation.

TABLE 2— Associations Between Psychosocial Syndemic Burden and Measures of Engagement in HIV Prevention Care: United States, February–October 2022

	HIV Test (Lifetime) (n = 2700 in Adjusted Analyses)[a]			PrEP Awareness (n = 885 in Adjusted Analyses)				PrEP Utilization (n = 9890 in Adjusted Analyses)			
	$n_{(event)}$ Yes/No[b]	AOR (95% CI)[c]	*P* for trend	$n_{(event)}$ Yes/No[b]	AOR (95% CI)[c]	*P* for Trend	Fully Adjusted OR (95% CI)[d]	$n_{(event)}$ Yes/No[b]	AOR (95% CI)[c]	*P* for Trend	Fully Adjusted OR (95% CI)[d]
Psychosocial Syndemic burden (Ref = 0 syndemic factors), no. syndemic factors	43/388	1 (Ref)	Linear: *P* < .001; Quadratic: *P* = .75; Cubic: *P* = .41	662/2066	1 (Ref)	Linear: *P* < .001; Quadratic: *P* = .36; Cubic: *P* = .30	1 (Ref)	10/2719	1 (Ref)	Linear: *P* < .001; Quadratic: *P* = .98; Cubic: *P* = .01	1 (Ref)
1	145/1072	1.42 (0.97, 2.09)		1456/4316	1.12 (1.00, 1.26)		1.08 (0.96, 1.21)	28/5745	1.42 (0.67, 2.97)		0.97 (0.45, 2.10)
2	149/723	2.55 (1.72, 3.78)		437/1063	1.26 (1.08, 1.47)		1.10 (0.93, 1.30)	30/1474	6.06 (2.87, 12.83)		3.25 (1.45, 7.31)
3	74/182	4.62 (2.94, 7.27)		134/190	2.09 (1.62, 2.69)		1.68 (1.27, 2.21)	25/298	23.86 (10.92, 52.15)		10.87 (4.57, 25.90)
4	32/50	7.25 (3.97, 13.25)		44/45	2.43 (1.53, 3.86)		1.71 (1.05, 2.81)	13/75	35.73 (13.40, 95.28)		10.15 (3.34, 30.79)
Depressive symptoms (yes/no)	247/1370 190/1015	0.88 (0.69, 1.11)		1385/4328 1330/3332	0.82 (0.74, 0.90)		0.82 (0.74, 0.90)	59/5647 47/4612	0.85 (0.55, 1.32)		0.90 (0.56, 1.44)
Sexual initiation (yes/no)	. . .	. . .		. . .	. . .		1.25 (1.09, 1.44)	. . .	. . .		1.68 (0.88, 3.20)
CAVS, 3 mo (yes/no)	. . .	. . .		. . .	. . .		0.96 (0.77, 1.19)	. . .	. . .		1.57 (0.84, 2.91)
No. of sexual partners	. . .	. . .		. . .	. . .		1.14 (1.04, 1.25)	. . .	. . .		1.28 (1.07, 1.53)

Note. AOR = adjusted odds ratio; CAVS = condomless anal or vaginal sex; CI = confidence interval; OR = odds ratio; PrEP = preexposure prophylaxis. All regression models considered psychosocial syndemic burden as a categorical variable and assessed linear, quadratic, and cubic trends.

[a]Among individuals who reported sexual initiation.

[b]Number of individuals reporting the outcome of interest (i.e., HIV testing, PrEP awareness, and PrEP use) and not reporting the outcome of interest by covariate level.

[c]Adjusted models controlled for age, race/ethnicity, gender identity, sex assigned at birth, and sexual orientation.

[d]Fully adjusted models controlled for sexual initiation, CAVS in the past 3 months, and number of sexual partners in addition to sociodemographics controlled for in adjusted models.

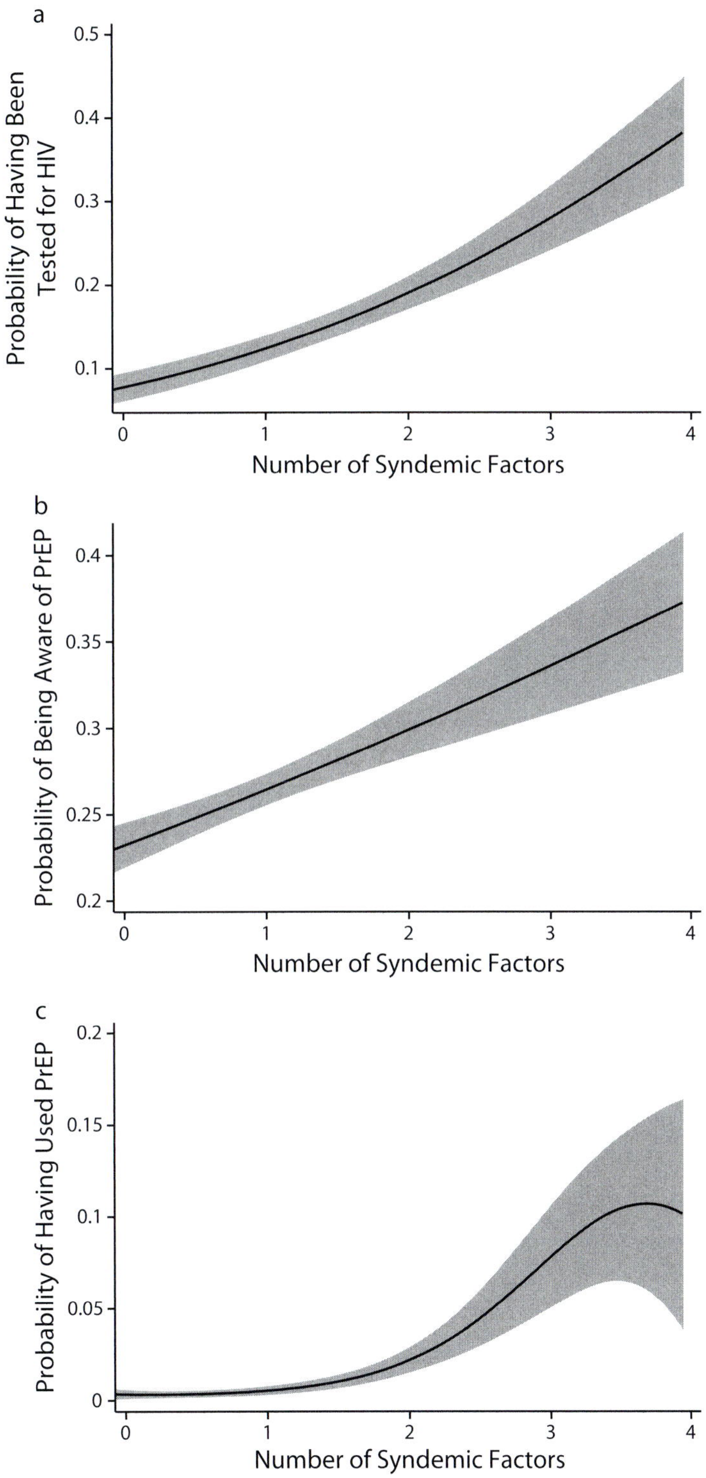

FIGURE 2— Number of Reported Psychosocial Syndemic Factors Based on Highest-Order Significant Polynomial Regression and Adjusted Predicted Probabilities of (a) HIV Testing, (b) Preexposure Prophylaxis (PrEP) Awareness, and (c) PrEP Utilization: United States, February–October 2022

Note. Parts a and b show fitted generalized linear models of predicted probabilities of HIV testing (among individuals who have had sex) and PrEP awareness (among all individuals) and psychosocial syndemic burden. Part c shows fitted cubic models of the relationship between predicted probabilities of PrEP utilization and psychosocial syndemic burden. Wide confidence intervals in part c reflect low prevalence of highest syndemic counts and PrEP utilization. In all models, psychosocial syndemic burden was considered as a continuous predictor. Adjusted models control for the effects of age, race/ethnicity, gender identity, sex assigned at birth, and sexual orientation.

CAVS was not associated with PrEP awareness or utilization (Table 2).

Additional post hoc analyses showed that race/ethnicity and gender identity significantly moderated the relationship between psychosocial syndemics and number of sexual partners ($P = .02$ and $P < .001$, respectively), such that this relationship was stronger among non-White and cisgender individuals (Supplemental Tables C–F; Supplemental Figures A and B, available as a supplement to the online version of this article at http://www.ajph.org).

Sensitivity Analysis

Findings from regression models in 50 imputed data sets showed consistent results regarding the directionality and magnitude of relationships between syndemic burden and our outcomes of interest (Supplemental Tables G–J, available as a supplement to the online version of this article at http://www.ajph.org).

DISCUSSION

Our study adds to the growing literature on syndemics and HIV prevention care among SGM youths. By examining linear and nonlinear relationships between syndemic factors and health outcomes, we have contributed to a more detailed understanding of the complex interplay between psychosocial syndemic factors and HIV risk and engagement in preventive care. Similar to previous studies,[10–12] we have shown a high prevalence of psychosocial syndemic factors among SGM youths. In our study, almost 20% of our sample reported 2 or more psychosocial syndemic factors, with anti-LGBTQ discrimination being particularly common, indicating that many SGM youths may need interventions to address multilevel psychosocial inequities.

As hypothesized, we identified a linear dose–response effect of psychosocial syndemic burden on sexual behaviors that may lead to HIV transmission. Several studies have shown an additive association between psychosocial syndemic factors and HIV risk behaviors in US adult[8,14] and youth[7,10,27] SGM populations. Our study adds to this body of work and demonstrates similar relationships in a large US sample of SGM individuals younger than 18 years, thus addressing a gap in the existing literature. We encourage further studies to explore mechanisms that could explain our post hoc findings of a stronger relationship between psychosocial syndemics among non-White and cisgender youths (e.g., intersectional discrimination and racism).

Unlike previous studies,[9,10,14] we found that the effects of depressive symptoms on sexual behaviors were different from those of the other syndemic factors; namely, depressive symptoms did not have a significant effect on sexual behaviors and were negatively associated with PrEP awareness. Because composite psychosocial syndemic burden variables assume that the individual effects of each syndemic factor are comparable,[17] we did not include depression as part of our composite index. Some of the studies that did include depression in counts of syndemic factors did not show depression to be individually associated with sexual behaviors.[7,8] Therefore, future syndemic studies should consider the effects of each syndemic factor on each other and on health outcomes individually before creating composite syndemic indicators.

There are several possible explanations for the different effects of depression symptoms and other syndemic factors. Depression symptoms may include decreased sexual drive[28] and are linked to social isolation and withdrawal,[29] which could limit opportunities for engaging in sexual behaviors and learning about PrEP from social networks. Further studies are needed to identify mediators between depression and sexual behaviors among SGM youths and to study effect modifiers of this relationship, which would help identify groups of youths for whom addressing depression symptoms may decrease HIV risk as well.

Contrary to our expectations, the psychosocial syndemic burden was associated with greater, rather than lower, engagement in HIV prevention care, a relationship that was only partially mediated by sexual risk behaviors. Although some studies have shown syndemic burden to be associated with lower HIV testing and decreased progression along the PrEP cascade,[15,30] others have, like our study, shown syndemic burden positively associated with PrEP engagement.[31–33] These results may reflect targeted efforts to engage the most at-risk individuals in PrEP care, resulting in higher PrEP awareness and utilization among individuals experiencing higher HIV risk. Importantly, predicted probabilities of PrEP utilization were low (< 15%) even for the highest levels of syndemic burden, indicating that additional efforts are still needed to reach youths experiencing multiple psychosocial problems and potentially at higher risk for HIV acquisition.

An important limitation of existing syndemics research is the dearth of studies examining synergism across syndemic factors.[19,34] Our study addressed this gap by examining nonlinear relationships between psychosocial syndemic burden and sexual behavior and HIV prevention outcomes. Specifically, we have shown synergistic polynomial relationships between syndemic burden and sexual behaviors and PrEP utilization. That is, as the burden of psychosocial syndemics increases, the number of sexual partners and the probability of reporting recent CAVS and PrEP utilization grow multiplicatively. These findings have implications for practice, as evidence of syndemic synergism suggests that multicomponent interventions addressing multiple syndemic factors at once may be more effective and efficient than intervening in individual factors. Indeed, existing HIV prevention interventions already incorporate components that address concomitant stigma and substance use, with promising results.[35,36] We believe that our study provides support for a combined approach in HIV prevention interventions, which should be further evaluated in future intervention studies.

Limitations

Our findings must be interpreted in light of the limitations of this study. First, as a cross-sectional study, our ability to infer causality and directionality is limited. Moreover, our study had a considerable amount of missing data, and although multiple imputations indicated that missingness did not affect findings significantly, this method relies on unverifiable assumptions. Additionally, our measure of binge drinking (5 drinks within a couple of hours) may have underestimated this behavior among individuals assigned female at birth, and sexual victimization considered only intercourse, which may have underestimated other forms of sexual victimization. Finally, despite our large sample, recruitment efforts relied on community-based organizations and online venues that may be frequented by SGM youths with greater access to affirming social groups and coping resources. Consequently, our findings may not be generalizable to all SGM youths in the United States.

Although Black and Latinx gay and bisexual men and transgender women are disproportionately vulnerable to acquiring HIV, most youths in our study were assigned female sex at birth and were White. Future studies should consider oversampling youths of color to allow more detailed descriptions of how psychosocial factors may affect HIV risk and engagement in care across racial and ethnic groups. These studies should also further examine the role of race, ethnicity, and gender identity as moderators of relationships between syndemics and health outcomes.

Conclusions

These limitations notwithstanding, our study highlights the need to address cooccurring syndemics of HIV risk and psychosocial problems among SGM youths. Multicomponent interventions addressing multilevel syndemic factors have been advocated in HIV research, yet empirical evidence for their improved performance, as opposed to separate interventions, has been relatively scarce. Further research should continue to examine synergism across syndemic factors to identify combinations of intervention components that result in the greatest impact. To that end, novel approaches such as the multiphase optimization strategy[37] may be particularly insightful for identifying specific intervention components that should be included in multicomponent interventions for improved effectiveness and efficiency. AJPH

ABOUT THE AUTHORS

Pablo K. Valente is with the Department of Allied Health Sciences, University of Connecticut, Waterbury. Raghavee Neupane was with the Boston University School of Public Health, Boston, MA, at the time of writing of this article. Lisa Eaton and Ryan J. Watson are with the Department of Human Development and Family Studies, University of Connecticut, Storrs.

CORRESPONDENCE

Correspondence should be sent to Pablo K. Valente, 99 East Main St, Room 114, Waterbury, CT 06702 (e-mail: pablo.valente@uconn.edu). Reprints can be ordered at https://www.ajph.org by clicking the "Reprints" link.

PUBLICATION INFORMATION

Full Citation: Valente PK, Neupane R, Eaton L, Watson RJ. Psychosocial syndemic burden, sexual behaviors, and engagement in HIV prevention care among sexual and gender minority youths: United States, 2022. *Am J Public Health*. 2024;114(9):892–902.

Acceptance Date: June 7, 2024.

DOI: https://doi.org/10.2105/AJPH.2024.307753

ORCID iD:

Pablo K. Valente https://orcid.org/0000-0002-2058-3472

CONTRIBUTORS

P. K. Valente performed the formal analyses. P. K. Valente, L. Eaton, and R. J. Watson conceptualized the study and developed the methodology. R. J. Watson acquired the funding. All authors contributed to writing the article.

ACKNOWLEDGMENTS

This work was supported by the National Institute on Drug Abuse, National Institutes of Health (NIH; grant K01DA047918, principal investigator: R. J. W.) and the National Institute on Minority Health and Health Disparities, NIH (grant R01MD015722-01S1).

The authors acknowledge the Human Rights Campaign Foundation for their partnership in data collection.

Note. The content of this article is solely the responsibility of the authors and does not necessarily represent the official views of the NIH.

CONFLICTS OF INTEREST

The authors have no conflicts of interests to report.

HUMAN PARTICIPANT PROTECTION

The University of Connecticut institutional review board reviewed and approved all study materials and procedures. Participants received US $5 for participation. All individuals provided informed electronic consent or assent, and we obtained a waiver of parental consent.

REFERENCES

1. Centers for Disease Control and Prevention. HIV surveillance report. May 2021. Available at: https://www.cdc.gov/hiv/pdf/library/reports/surveillance/cdc-hiv-surveillance-report-2018-updated-vol-32.pdf. Accessed June 26, 2024.
2. Centers for Disease Control and Prevention. Sexual risk behavior differences among sexual minority high school students—United States, 2015 and 2017. *MMWR Morb Mortal Wkly Rep*. 2018; 67(36):1007–1011. https://doi.org/10.15585/mmwr.mm6736a3
3. Centers for Disease Control and Prevention. Prescription opioid misuse and use of alcohol and other substances among high school students—Youth Risk Behavior Survey, United States, 2019. *MMWR Suppl*. 2020;69(1):38–46. https://doi.org/10.15585/mmwr.su6901a5
4. Centers for Disease Control and Prevention. HIV testing, linkage to HIV medical care, and interviews for partner services among youths—61 health department jurisdictions, United States, Puerto Rico, and the US Virgin Islands, 2015. *MMWR Morb Mortal Wkly Rep*. 2017;66(24): 629–635. https://doi.org/10.15585/mmwr.mm6624a2
5. Barocas JA, Gai MJ, Nurani A, Bagley SM, Hadland SE. Initiation of HIV pre-exposure prophylaxis among youth in the United States, 2015–2018. *AIDS Care*. 2023;35(3):431–436. https://doi.org/10.1080/09540121.2022.2067318
6. Singer M. A dose of drugs, a touch of violence, a case of AIDS: conceptualizing the SAVA syndemic. *Free Inq Creat Sociol*. 1996;24(2):13–24.
7. Teixeira da Silva D, Bouris A, Voisin D, Hotton A, Brewer R, Schneider J. Social networks moderate the syndemic effect of psychosocial and structural factors on HIV risk among young black transgender women and men who have sex with men. *AIDS Behav*. 2020;24(1):192–205. https://doi.org/10.1007/s10461-019-02575-9
8. Mimiaga MJ, O'Cleirigh C, Biello KB, et al. The effect of psychosocial syndemic production on 4-year HIV incidence and risk behavior in a large cohort of sexually active men who have sex with men. *J Acquir Immune Defic Syndr*. 2015;68(3): 329–336. https://doi.org/10.1097/QAI.0000000000000475
9. Mustanski B, Phillips G, Ryan DT, Swann G, Kuhns L, Garofalo R. Prospective effects of a syndemic on HIV and STI incidence and risk behaviors in a cohort of young men who have sex with men. *AIDS Behav*. 2017;21(3):845–857. https://doi.org/10.1007/s10461-016-1607-3
10. Mimiaga MJ, Hughto JMW, Biello KB, et al. Longitudinal analysis of syndemic psychosocial problems predicting HIV risk behavior among a multicity prospective cohort of sexually active young transgender women in the United States. *J Acquir Immune Defic Syndr*. 2019;81(2):184–192. https://doi.org/10.1097/QAI.0000000000002009
11. Pellicane MJ, Ciesla JA. Temporal trends in rates of depression, anxiety, and suicidality among cisgender sexual minority and heterosexual college students. *Psychol Sex Orientat Gend Divers*. 2023;10(4):560–574. https://doi.org/10.1037/sgd0000563s
12. Fish JN, Bishop MD, Russell ST. Developmental differences in sexual orientation and gender identity–related substance use disparities: findings from population-based data. *J Adolesc Health*. 2021;68(6):1162–1169. https://doi.org/10.1016/j.jadohealth.2020.10.023
13. Meyer IH. Prejudice, social stress, and mental health in lesbian, gay, and bisexual populations: conceptual issues and research evidence. *Psychol Bull*. 2003;129(5):674–697. https://doi.org/10.1037/0033-2909.129.5.674
14. Harkness A, Bainter SA, O'Cleirigh C, Albright C, Mayer KH, Safren SA. Longitudinal effects of syndemics on HIV-positive sexual minority men's sexual health behaviors. *Arch Sex Behav*. 2019; 48(4):1159–1170. https://doi.org/10.1007/s10508-018-1329-x
15. Blashill AJ, Brady JP, Rooney BM, et al. Syndemics and the PrEP cascade: results from a sample of young Latino men who have sex with men. *Arch Sex Behav*. 2020;49(1):125–135. https://doi.org/10.1007/s10508-019-01470-7
16. Myers K, Li T, Baum M, Ibanez G, Fennie K. The individual, interactive, and syndemic effect of substance use, depression, education, and ethnicity on retention in HIV care. *Int J STD AIDS*. 2021;32(2):184–193. https://doi.org/10.1177/0956462419890727
17. Tsai AC, Venkataramani AS. Syndemics and health disparities: a methodological note. *AIDS Behav*. 2016;20(2):423–430. https://doi.org/10.1007/s10461-015-1260-2
18. Singer M, Clair S. Syndemics and public health: reconceptualizing disease in bio-social context. *Med Anthropol Q*. 2003;17(4):423–441. https://doi.org/10.1525/maq.2003.17.4.423
19. Tsai AC, Burns BFO. Syndemics of psychosocial problems and HIV risk: a systematic review of empirical tests of the disease interaction concept. *Soc Sci Med*. 2015;139:26–35. https://doi.org/10.1016/j.socscimed.2015.06.024
20. Tomori C, McFall AM, Solomon SS, et al. Is there synergy in syndemics? Psychosocial conditions and sexual risk among men who have sex with men in India. *Soc Sci Med*. 2018;206:110–116. https://doi.org/10.1016/j.socscimed.2018.03.032
21. Bulled N. A new approach to measuring the synergy in a syndemic: revisiting the SAVA syndemic among urban MSM in the United States. *Glob Public Health*. 2022;17(9):2070–2080. https://doi.org/10.1080/17441692.2021.1974513
22. Wirtz AL, Burns PA, Poteat T, et al. Abuse in the continua: HIV prevention and care outcomes and syndemic conditions associated with intimate partner violence among Black gay and bisexual men in the Southern United States. *AIDS Behav*. 2022;26(11):3761–3774. https://doi.org/10.1007/s10461-022-03705-6
23. Bhardwaj A, Comins CA, Guddera V, et al. Prevalence of depression, syndemic factors and their impact on viral suppression among female sex workers living with HIV in eThekwini, South Africa. *BMC Womens Health*. 2023;23(1):232. https://doi.org/10.1186/s12905-023-02392-2
24. Halkitis PN, Kapadia F, Bub KL, Barton S, Moreira AD, Stults CB. A longitudinal investigation of syndemic conditions among young gay, bisexual, and other MSM: the P18 Cohort Study. *AIDS Behav*. 2015;19(6):970–980. https://doi.org/10.1007/s10461-014-0892-y
25. Watson RJ, Caba AE, Lawrence SE, et al. Examining mental health and bullying concerns at the intersection of sexuality, gender, race, and ethnicity among a national sample of sexual and gender diverse youth. *LGBT Health*. 2024;11(1): 20–27. https://doi.org/10.1089/lgbt.2023.0072
26. Kroenke K, Spitzer RL, Williams JB. The Patient Health Questionnaire-2: validity of a two-item depression screener. *Med Care*. 2003;41(11): 1284–1292. https://doi.org/10.1097/01.MLR.0000093487.78664.3C
27. Brennan J, Kuhns LM, Johnson AK, et al. Syndemic theory and HIV-related risk among young transgender women: the role of multiple, co-occurring health problems and social marginalization. *Am J Public Health*. 2012;102(9): 1751–1757. https://doi.org/10.2105/AJPH.2011.300433
28. Laurent SM, Simons AD. Sexual dysfunction in depression and anxiety: conceptualizing sexual dysfunction as part of an internalizing dimension. *Clin Psychol Rev*. 2009;29(7):573–585. https://doi.org/10.1016/j.cpr.2009.06.007
29. Rueger SY, Malecki CK, Pyun Y, Aycock C, Coyle S. A meta-analytic review of the association between perceived social support and depression in childhood and adolescence. *Psychol Bull*. 2016;142(10):1017–1067. https://doi.org/10.1037/bul0000058
30. Turpin R, Slopen N, Boekeloo B, Dallal C, Chen S, Dyer T. Testing a syndemic index of psychosocial and structural factors associated with HIV testing among Black men. *J Health Care Poor Underserved*. 2020;31(1):455–470. https://doi.org/10.1353/hpu.2020.0033
31. Chandler CJ, Bukowski LA, Matthews DD, et al. Understanding the impact of a syndemic on the use of pre-exposure prophylaxis in a community-based sample of behaviorally PrEP-eligible BMSM in the United States. *AIDS Care*. 2020;32(5):551–556. https://doi.org/10.1080/09540121.2019.1659921
32. Willie TC, Kershaw TS, Blackstock O, et al. Racial and ethnic differences in women's HIV risk and attitudes towards pre-exposure prophylaxis (PrEP) in the context of the substance use, violence, and depression syndemic. *AIDS Care*. 2021;33(2):219–228. https://doi.org/10.1080/09540121.2020.1762067
33. Kuhns LM, Perloff J, Johnson AK, et al. A cross-sectional analysis of psychosocial and structural barriers and facilitators associated with PrEP use among a sample of transgender women in Chicago, IL. *AIDS Res Ther*. 2023;20(1):24. https://doi.org/10.1186/s12981-023-00516-0
34. Singer M, Bulled N, Ostrach B. Whither syndemics? Trends in syndemics research, a review 2015–2019. *Glob Public Health*. 2020;15(7):943–955. https://doi.org/10.1080/17441692.2020.1724317
35. Garofalo R, Kuhns LM, Reisner SL, Biello K, Mimiaga MJ. Efficacy of an empowerment-based, group-delivered HIV prevention intervention for young transgender women: the Project LifeSkills randomized clinical trial. *JAMA Pediatr*. 2018;172(10): 916–923. https://doi.org/10.1001/jamapediatrics.2018.1799
36. Bogart LM, Barreras JL, Gonzalez A, et al. Pilot randomized controlled trial of an intervention to improve coping with intersectional stigma and medication adherence among HIV-positive Latinx sexual minority men. *AIDS Behav*. 2021;25(6): 1647–1660. https://doi.org/10.1007/s10461-020-03081-z
37. Collins LM, Kugler KC, Gwadz MV. Optimization of multicomponent behavioral and biobehavioral interventions for the prevention and treatment of HIV/AIDS. *AIDS Behav*. 2016;20(suppl 1): S197–S214. https://doi.org/10.1007/s10461-015-1145-4

The History of US Menstrual Health, School Nurses, and the Future of Menstrual Health Equity

Sadie Bergen, MA, MPhil, Erin D. Maughan, RN, PhD, MS, PHNA-BC, Karen E. Johnson, RN, PhD, Robin Cogan, RN, MEd, NCSN, Molly Secor, PhD, MS, BSN, and Marni Sommer, RN, DrPH, MSN

See also Tobbell, p. 849.

In the United States, adolescents suffer from inadequate menstrual health, meaning that adolescents are unprepared for menarche, lack the practical resources they need to comfortably and confidently manage menstruation, and receive inadequate health education and care for menstrual pain and disorders. In this article, we provide a historical analysis of the role of school nurses in addressing menstruation from the early 20th century up to the present day. We contextualize the current realities of school nursing and menstrual health education and clinical support. We argue that the decentralized US school system, a cultural aversion to open discussion about menstruation, and the outsized influence of commercial menstrual product manufacturers have hampered the ability of school nurses to deliver menstrual health education along with menstrual health support. Finally, we discuss implications for today's schooling experiences as well as recommendations for how to support school nurses in aligning our national approach to menstrual health toward the public health perspective of menstrual equity. (*Am J Public Health*. 2024;114(9):903–908. https://doi.org/10.2105/AJPH.2024.307705)

In recent years, research and public advocacy have brought attention to disparities in menstrual health in the United States, particularly among adolescents. "Menstrual health" is a holistic term that includes access to menstrual education, menstrual products, adequate toilet facilities, health care for menstrual pain and menstrual disorders, and freedom from stigma and discrimination.[1] Globally, menstrual health has been incorporated into a public health paradigm, with research demonstrating that poor menstrual health and hygiene can negatively impact students' educational experiences and their health and well-being.[2] The limited available evidence from the United States suggests that students here also suffer from inadequate menstrual health. Many are unprepared for menarche, lack the practical resources they need to comfortably and confidently manage menstruation, and receive inadequate health education and care for menstrual pain and disorders. For example, a 2017 systematic review of the pubertal experiences of low-income girls indicated that many girls felt that the menstruation information provided by schools was inaccurate, negative, and came too late.[3] More recent research conducted with US adolescent girls and educators shores up these findings.[4–10]

State-level legislative efforts have primarily focused on improving "menstrual equity" in US schools by mandating free menstrual products in public school bathrooms.[11,12] Such legislation aims to combat period poverty, which has been tied to missed school days and worse academic performance.[4] To date, there has not been systematic evaluation of the implementation of these policies, and while menstrual product access is a crucial component of menstrual health, the effort to promote menstrual equity in schools must address all dimensions of menstrual health to truly impact population health. Addressing menstrual health comprehensively would encompass provision of menstrual education and the delivery of menstrual health care as needed in the school environment by adequately trained and resourced school nurses. In this essay, we aim to provide a historical analysis of the role of school nurses in addressing menstruation from the early 20th century up to the present day and discuss implications for today's schooling

AJPH September 2024, Vol. 114, No. 9

experiences as well as recommendations for how to support school nurses in establishing an equity-focused national approach to menstrual health.

Timely, accurate, and appropriately delivered menstruation education has the potential to improve menstrual health literacy among all students, combat menstrual stigma, and direct adolescents to appropriate care when needed. School nurses have been identified as particularly well suited to provide menstrual health education and care.[5,6,13] They are trusted members of the school community and bring medical expertise to care for and refer students as needed. Yet a review of the history of school nurses and their relationship to menstrual health reveals how the decentralized US school system, a cultural aversion to open discussion about menstruation, and the outsized influence of commercial menstrual product manufacturers have hampered the ability of school nurses to deliver menstrual health education and menstrual health support.

HISTORY OF SCHOOL NURSES IN MENSTRUAL EDUCATION AND CARE

School nurses have been supporting and educating menstruating students since the early 20th century, when the profession was founded and US adolescents began attending school in large numbers.[14,15] The broad scope of early school nursing practice included physical examinations, care coordination, home visitation, and health education.[14] According to a 1918 school nursing handbook, nurses were "constantly being called upon to give information" to girls about "matters of personal and social hygiene."[16(p5)] The handbook identified a lack of health literacy among the student population yet constrained nurses' ability to take action, instructing them to share information only with the consent of the student's mother, "who is the natural instructor of the girl in such intimate matters."[16(p52)] Menstruation, including guidance for those reaching menarche, was primarily relegated to the private sphere alongside other subjects related to sex and sexuality even as reformers argued vociferously about whether and how they should be incorporated into public school education.[17,18]

In communicating a sense that menstruation was too "intimate" for school while not adequately addressing the gap in girls' knowledge about menstrual health, the 1918 manual left a void that menstrual product companies such as Kimberly-Clark enthusiastically filled. In 1921, Kimberly-Clark created Kotex, the first disposable menstrual product. To convince women and girls that disposable pads were superior to homemade cloth pads and reusable sanitary belts, the company began producing educational pamphlets for female audiences, including young girls, mothers, and working women.[17] This effort extended into classrooms, with Kimberly-Clark providing schools with materials (including menstrual products) that could be distributed directly to students by school nurses, professionals who were identified by Kimberly-Clark as important gatekeepers to the company's joint educational and commercial mission.[19]

By the 1940s, menstrual education (and sex education in general) became more widespread in the school setting alongside a rising tide of interest in promoting healthy adolescent development in the United States.[20] These classes were often organized by the principal and school nurse and aimed to provide up-to-date scientific information about the physiology of menstruation as well as cultivate a positive attitude toward the social dimensions of growing up, including the normative heterosexual expectations around marriage, sex, and family life.[20]

The decentralized nature of US education in the 1940s meant that menstrual health programs were implemented (as one component of sex education and family life curricula) at the district level through the efforts and cooperation of parents, educators, and health professionals.[20] Decentralization also fostered racial inequities across the school system by allowing educational resources, including health education and school health services, to fall along lines set by structural racism in its many forms, from legally segregated schools in the Jim Crow South to the neighborhood segregation and economic inequality of schools across the country.[21]

In the absence of Department of Education curricula for health educators or a mandate for school nurses, most menstrual education took the form of commercially produced materials. Commercial health education films were a phenomenon of the mid-20th century, covering subjects of public health concern from tuberculosis to venereal disease. In 1946, Kimberly-Clark expanded their educational offerings with the release of *The Story of Menstruation*, an educational film produced in collaboration with Disney. The film paired a truncated explanation of the science of menstruation alongside a sunny, animated narrative of a young, White girl for whom menarche inspired daydreams about a future of marriage and babies, thus setting a normative standard of Whiteness and heterosexuality shaped by the racialized social values of the time.[19,20] Notably absent from the film were details about the other dimensions of puberty, such as bodily changes and hormonal fluctuations. Rather, the ideology of the film seems to have been to infuse a "hygienic imperative" of menstrual self-care into an ideological framework of heteronormativity.[19,22] Outside of Kimberly-Clark and Disney representatives, the film had sign-off from the medical establishment: it was reviewed by a gynecologist before its release and received a positive reception from the American Medical Association.[23]

School nurses served as a conduit between corporate menstrual education materials and their student audiences and provided direct clinical care for students experiencing menstruation in school. In both roles, their resources for providing education and care were shaped by the times they were living in. School nursing texts from the mid-20th century encouraged nurses to normalize menstruation and, as a 1949 manual put it, "avoid the formation of a mental attitude of invalidism in connection with the menstrual period,"[24(p61)] advice that must be read with an awareness of the longer history of assumptions that menstruation made women weak and unsuited for equal educational opportunities to men. Guidance was also shaped by the normative gender roles of the mid-20th century: for instance, the nursing manual explained that menstrual pain may be an expression of "marital unhappiness in the home from which the pupil comes, an overly solicitous mother, or the rejection of the 'woman role' in life on the part of the pupil."[24(p62)] Educational materials were also a reflection of the limited biomedical understandings of menstruation and menstrual disorders at midcentury.[25] For example, a school nurse looking for guidance on how much physical activity to recommend for menstruating students in the 1940s or 1950s would have encountered conflicting information—from advice that girls "not 'jiggle' their uteri too much"[17(p92)] to reassurances that activity during menstruation was "rarely contraindicated."[24(p74)]

School nurses have consistently been expected to deliver menstrual health education and clinical care without adequate preparation with which to do so independently. By the late 20th century, multiple paths to nursing qualification had opened up, and states implemented different models of school nurse certification, including a range of expectations and responsibilities for health education.[26,27] A 1960 article in *Nursing Outlook* reported that nursing school did not prepare future school nurses to teach adolescents about menstruation.[28] Thus, films like *The Story of Menstruation* were a pragmatic and popular tool that allowed school nurses to deal with the subject. Several school nurses are quoted in Kimberly-Clark's *Practical Guide for Teaching Menstrual Hygiene* praising the quality of the company's film and written materials. Voicing a perspective common at the time, one school nurse noted in the pamphlet that "our school system . . . believes that teaching on menstruation belongs in the home. Therefore, all I do is try to help mothers so that they can help their daughters."[29(p10)] The substance of these commercial materials was not necessarily inaccurate in their descriptions of menstrual cycle physiology,[30] but as feminist analyses of these materials began to point out in the 1970s, they were incomplete and biased toward a particular approach to menstrual hygiene that emphasized concealment and overlooked the embodied experience of menstruation for adolescents.[31]

In the 1980s, Kimberly-Clark replaced *The Story of Menstruation* with a new film, *Julie's Story*, which reflected the influences of the feminist women's health movement[22] by centering the experience of menstruation for an individual girl. The film was developed with substantial input from an advisory board, including the executive director of the National Association of School Nurses (NASN) and three local school nurses. *Julie's Story* and its accompanying educational materials were sent directly to school nurse offices and distributed to state health education officials around the country. At the same time, Procter & Gamble developed a menstrual education program that included a film, educational guides, and samples of the brand's pads. The program was also evaluated and endorsed by the NASN. In fact, in 1989, program materials were sent to school nurses with an accompanying letter from the NASN president, citing it as an exemplar of puberty education.[23] According to historian Dan Guadagnolo, by the late 20th century, commercial menstrual education had become the norm in the United States, a trend that continues into the present day.[19] Unfortunately we do not know how these materials were distributed around the country or to what extent they were incorporated into school curricula.

In 1995, a small survey of 39 school nurses found that the majority (85%) were responsible for teaching about menstruation in their schools. However, this responsibility was only sporadically supported by dedicated financial or pedagogical resources. As the survey authors wrote in their conclusion, "more attention needs to be paid to the resources [nurses] have available."[32(p682)] In 2022, a survey of elementary school nurses found that the majority of them taught menstrual health and were interested in learning about the best way to impart this critical information to their students.[24] A range of educators, including physical education teachers and science teachers, has historically been assigned the role of educating young people about menstruation and puberty. But even if they are not the primary health education instructors, health education falls within the school nurse's scope of practice, and the role is uniquely positioned to provide one-on-one education to students.[33] The lack of consistent school nurses at some schools because of resource limitations can negatively impact the ability of teachers to collaborate with them on imparting menstrual health and management guidance to students.[5]

CURRENT REALITIES OF SCHOOL NURSES AND MENSTRUAL EQUITY

Constraints on school nursing resources, the decentralization of US schools, and the association of menstrual health education with sex education—the latter of which may be restricted in some schools—pose significant barriers to the delivery of comprehensive menstrual health education and care in schools. A key challenge today is that school nurses across the country are underfunded and underresourced to deliver the care they have been trained to provide.[34] The inadequate fiscal prioritization for school nurses has meant that, for many years, public school districts around the country, particularly those in low-resource communities, lack sufficient school nursing staff.[34,35] Menstrual periods do not only show up one day per week, and so support and care for young people who may be managing excessive menstruation- or endometriosis-related pain or bleeding is difficult to provide without more regular school nurse staff.[36] In addition, the ability of school nurses to provide menstrual education is challenged by the more complex health needs of the US school-going population from elementary to high school: rates of diabetes mellitus, attention-deficit/hyperactivity disorder, asthma, and mental health concerns have all increased over time.[37] In recent years, the demands of the COVID-19 pandemic have further swelled the weekly work burden on school nurses.[38] These dynamics severely hinder the ability of school nurses to build the trusting relationships with students needed to provide menstrual care or to deliver menstrual health education.

While the growing global menstrual health agenda within public health has brought recognition that menstrual health should not be relegated to the private sphere, there is no shared national mandate for menstrual education in the United States. While state standards for health education about topics like nutrition and body systems are common, only a handful of states have standards for menstrual health.[8] A recent hearing on menstrual equity in New York City schools revealed that a protocol does not exist for a girl's first period happening in school, despite protocols existing for nosebleeds and stomach aches.[39] This absence of guidance at every level contributes both to the profound neglect of menstrual health literacy as central to population health and to the underuse of adequately trained and resourced school nurses to meet this need. The Title IX legislation released for public comment by the federal Department of Education in 2022 did not have a single mention of the word "menstruation," which would suggest that this gap may persist if not addressed by strong advocacy to make the connections between menstrual health and gender equity in schools.[40] School nurses do not provide classroom health education in every state or district because of the heterogeneity of health education standards and certifications, a status quo that only reinforces the need for strong federal guidelines about the provision of menstrual health education and support that could be adapted by school nurses for their local conditions.

A final challenge is that social and political influences continue to shape what is taught in US schools, as in many countries around the world. Parents and caregivers have an important role to play in supporting and educating their children as they develop into young adults, including having a trust in the educational system. However, this also means that menstruation education is often coupled with the delivery of sex education, which in most states can be opted out of upon parental request (sex education requires "opt-in" parental consent in four states).[41] Something as fundamental and basic as menstruation, a natural part of the child developmental experience for half the population of young people in our schools today, is central to the health-related education that should be provided. The stakes of such education are high: research from across the United States indicates that many girls are not prepared for their first period, and experience fear, shame, and anxiety when they bleed for the first time.[4] Yet parents and caregivers are often uncomfortable talking to their children about menstruation.[5] School nurses, armed with menstrual health standards in schools and working in collaboration with health educators, could fundamentally address this challenge. They are also positioned to provide the menstrual health care that young people need for both normal menstrual experiences and menstrual disorders throughout their schooling experiences. As the average age of menarche in the United States is now 11.9 years, school nurses prepared and resourced for supporting menstrual health education and care are essential from elementary school onward through high school.[42] AJPH

ABOUT THE AUTHORS

Sadie Bergen and Marni Sommer are with the Department of Sociomedical Sciences at Columbia University Mailman School of Public Health, New York, NY. Erin D. Maughan is with the George Mason University College of Public Health, Fairfax, VA. Karen E. Johnson is with the University of Texas at Austin School of Nursing. Robin Cogan is with Rutgers School of Nursing and is a school nurse in the Camden City School District, Camden, NJ. Molly Secor is with Montana State University Mark and Robyn Jones College of Nursing, Bozeman.

CORRESPONDENCE

Correspondence should be sent to Sadie Bergen, MA, MPhil, Department of Sociomedical Sciences, Mailman School of Public Health, 722 W 168th St, New York, NY 10032 (e-mail: srb2161@columbia.edu). Reprints can be ordered at https://www.ajph.org by clicking the "Reprints" link.

PUBLICATION INFORMATION

Full Citation: Bergen S, Maughan ED, Johnson KE, Cogan R, Secor M, Sommer M. The history of US menstrual health, school nurses, and the future of menstrual health equity. *Am J Public Health.* 2024;114(9):903–908.

Acceptance Date: April 17, 2024.

DOI: https://doi.org/10.2105/AJPH.2024.307705

ORCID iDs:

Sadie Bergen https://orcid.org/0000-0002-3939-7645

Marni Sommer https://orcid.org/0000-0001-7442-9270

CONTRIBUTORS

S. Bergen, M. Sommer, E. D. Maughan, K. E. Johnson, and R. Cogan conceptualized the piece. Initial writing was done by S. Bergen and M. Sommer. All authors reviewed and contributed substantive edits on multiple versions of the article. All authors have read and agreed to the published version of the article.

ACKNOWLEDGMENTS

Funding for this research was provided in part by the Sid & Helaine Lerner Menstrual Hygiene Management Faculty Support Fund.

CONFLICTS OF INTEREST

The authors report that they have no conflicts of interest.

REFERENCES

1. Hennegan J, Winkler IT, Bobel C, et al. Menstrual health: a definition for policy, practice, and research. *Sex Reprod Health Matters.* 2021;29(1):1911618. https://doi.org/10.1080/26410397.2021.1911618
2. Sommer M, Caruso BA, Sahin M, et al. A time for global action: addressing girls' menstrual hygiene management needs in schools. *PLoS Med.* 2016; 13(2):e1001962. https://doi.org/10.1371/journal.pmed.1001962
3. Herbert AC, Ramirez AM, Lee G, et al. Puberty experiences of low-income girls in the United States: a systematic review of qualitative literature from 2000 to 2014. *J Adolesc Health.* 2017; 60(4):363–379. https://doi.org/10.1016/j.jadohealth.2016.10.008
4. Cotropia CA. Menstruation management in United States schools and implications for attendance, academic performance, and health. *Womens Reprod Health (Phila).* 2019;6(4):289–305. https://doi.org/10.1080/23293691.2019.1653575
5. Schmitt ML, Hagstrom C, Nowara A, et al. The intersection of menstruation, school and family: experiences of girls growing up in urban cities in the USA. *Int J Adolesc Youth.* 2021;26(1):94–109. https://doi.org/10.1080/02673843.2020.1867207
6. Secor-Turner M, Huseth-Zosel A, Ostlund R. Menstruation experiences of middle and high school students in the Midwest: a pilot study. *J Sch Nurs.* 2022;38(6):504–510. https://doi.org/10.1177/1059840520974234
7. Sebert Kuhlmann A, Teni MT, Key R, Billingsley C. Period product insecurity, school absenteeism, and use of school resources to obtain period products among high school students in St. Louis, Missouri. *J Sch Nurs.* 2024;40(3):329–335. https://doi.org/10.1177/10598405211069601
8. Sebert Kuhlmann A, Hunter E, Wall LL, Boyko M, Teni MT. State standards for menstrual hygiene education in US schools. *J Sch Health.* 2022;92(4): 418–420. https://doi.org/10.1111/josh.13135
9. Schmitt ML, Gruer C, Hagstrom C, et al. "It always gets pushed aside:" qualitative perspectives on puberty and menstruation education in USA schools. *Front Reprod Health.* 2022;4:1018217. https://doi.org/10.3389/frph.2022.1018217
10. Schmitt ML, Hagstrom C, Gruer C, et al. "Girls may bleed through pads because of demerits": adolescent girls' experiences with menstruation and school bathrooms in the USA. *J Adolesc Res.* 2024;39(2):511–536. https://doi.org/10.1177/07435584221139342
11. Francis L, Meraj S, Konduru D, Perrin EM. An update on state legislation supporting menstrual hygiene products in US schools: a legislative review, policy report, and recommendations for school nurse leadership. *J Sch Nurs.* 2023;39(6): 536–541. https://doi.org/10.1177/1059840522 1131012
12. Schmitt ML, Booth K, Sommer M. A policy for addressing menstrual equity in schools: a case study from New York City, USA. *Front Reprod Health.* 2022;3:725805.
13. Sebert Kuhlmann A, Palovick KA, Teni MT, Hunter E. Period product resources and needs in schools: a statewide survey of Missouri's school nurses. *J Sch Health.* 2023;93(7):557–564. https://doi.org/10.1111/josh.13326
14. Hawkins JW, Hayes ER, Corliss CP. School nursing in America—1902–1994: a return to public health nursing. *Public Health Nurs.* 1994;11(6):416–425. https://doi.org/10.1111/j.1525-1446.1994.tb00208.x
15. Mintz S. *Huck's Raft: A History of American Childhood.* Cambridge, MA: Belknap Press of Harvard University Press; 2004.
16. Kelly HW, Bradshaw MC. *A Handbook for School Nurses.* The Macmillan Company; 1918. Available at: http://hdl.loc.gov/loc.gdc/scd0001.00294639883. Accessed September 11, 2022.
17. Freidenfelds L. *The Modern Period: Menstruation in Twentieth-Century America.* Baltimore, MD: Johns Hopkins University Press; 2009.
18. Sommer M, Hirsch JS, Nathanson C, Parker RG. Comfortably, safely, and without shame: defining menstrual hygiene management as a public health issue. *Am J Public Health.* 2015;105(7):1302–1311. https://doi.org/10.2105/AJPH.2014.302525
19. Guadagnolo D. "The miracle of you": women's sex education and the marketing of Kotex. *Modern American History.* 2020;3(2-3):133–151. https://doi.org/10.1017/mah.2020.13
20. Freeman SK. *Sex Goes to School: Girls and Sex Education Before the 1960s.* Champaign, IL: University of Illinois Press; 2008.
21. Lassiter MD. Schools and housing in metropolitan history: an introduction. *J Urban Hist.* 2012; 38(2):195–204. https://doi.org/10.1177/00961 44211427111
22. Brumberg JJ. "Something happens to girls": menarche and the emergence of the modern American hygienic imperative. *J Hist Sex.* 1993;4(1):99–127.
23. Kennard ME. *The Corporation in the Classroom: The Struggles Over Meanings of Menstrual Education in Sponsored Films, 1947–1983.* PhD dissertation. The University of Wisconsin–Madison; 1989. Available at: http://www.proquest.com/docview/303806363/abstract/FDCCF43B14864A29PQ/1. Accessed March 29, 2022.
24. University of the State of New York. *The Work of the School Nurse-Teacher.* 1949. Available at: https://catalog.hathitrust.org/Record/100711625. Accessed March 31, 2022.
25. Clancy K. *Period: The Real Story of Menstruation.* Princeton, NJ: Princeton University Press; 2023. https://doi.org/10.1515/9780691246826
26. Thurber F, Berry B, Cameron ME. The role of school nursing in the United States. *J Pediatr Health Care.* 1991;5(3):135–140. https://doi.org/10.1016/0891-5245(91)90023-J
27. Anderson NE. The historical development of American nursing education. *Occup Health Nurs.* 1981;29(10):14–26. https://doi.org/10.1177/216507998102901002
28. Miller E. Adolescence: on the road to womanhood. *Nurs Outlook.* 1960;8:505–507.
29. Kimberly-Clark Corporation. *A Practical Guide for Teaching Menstrual Hygiene.* 1961. Available at: http://digitalwolfgram.widener.edu/digital/collection/p16069coll34/id/22. Accessed April 7, 2022.

30. Erchull MJ, Chrisler JC, Gorman JA, Johnston-Robledo I. Education and advertising: a content analysis of commercially produced booklets about menstruation. *J Early Adolesc.* 2002;22(4): 455–474. https://doi.org/10.1177/027243102237192
31. Whisnant L, Brett E, Zegans L. Implicit messages concerning menstruation in commercial educational materials prepared for young adolescent girls. *Am J Psychiatry.* 1975;132(8):815–820. https://doi.org/10.1176/ajp.132.8.815
32. Swenson IE, Foster B, Asay M. Menstruation, menarche, and sexuality in the public school curriculum: school nurses' perceptions. *Adolescence.* 1995;30(119):677–683.
33. National Association of School Nurses. Framework for 21st century school nursing practice: National Association of School Nurses. *NASN Sch Nurse.* 2016;31(1):45–53. https://doi.org/10.1177/1942602X15618644
34. Morse BL, Anderson L, Combe LG, Delack S, Ondeck L, Homme CUS. School nursing job analysis [erratum in *J Sch Nurs.* 2022;38(3):318]. *J Sch Nurs.* 2022;38(2):126–137. https://doi.org/10.1177/1059840520930075
35. Willgerodt MA, Brock DM, Maughan ED. Public school nursing practice in the United States. *J Sch Nurs.* 2018;34(3):232–244. https://doi.org/10.1177/1059840517752456
36. Hewitt G. Dysmenorrhea and endometriosis: diagnosis and management in adolescents. *Clin Obstet Gynecol.* 2020;63(3):536–543. https://doi.org/10.1097/GRF.0000000000000540
37. McCabe EM, Jameson BE, Strauss SM. School nurses matter: relationship between school nurse employment policies and chronic health condition policies in US school districts. *J Sch Nurs.* 2022;38(5):467–477. https://doi.org/10.1177/1059840520973413
38. Galemore CA, Marion S, Moran Fossile K, O'Toole S, Ragan K, Robertson B. Leading during a pandemic: a school nurse administrator roundtable. *NASN Sch Nurse.* 2022;37(3):155–164. https://doi.org/10.1177/1942602X221084069
39. The New York City Council. Meeting of Committee on Women and Gender Equity on 9/18/2023 at 10:00 AM. Available at: https://legistar.council.nyc.gov/MeetingDetail.aspx?ID=1115447&GUID=F5478D25-968E-4F77-8F00-DBFAA25854668&Options=info%7C&Search=. Accessed November 17, 2023.
40. US Department of Education. The US Department of Education releases proposed changes to Title IX regulations, invites public comment. June 23, 2022. Available at: https://www.ed.gov/news/press-releases/us-department-education-releases-proposed-changes-title-ix-regulations-invites-public-comment. Accessed November 15, 2023.
41. Garg N, Volerman A. A national analysis of state policies on lesbian, gay, bisexual, transgender, and questioning/queer inclusive sex education. *J Sch Health.* 2021;91(2):164–175. https://doi.org/10.1111/josh.12987
42. Martinez GM. Trends and patterns in menarche in the United States: 1995. *Natl Health Stat Rep.* 2020(146):1–12.

Likelihood of COVID-19 Outbreaks in US Immigration and Customs Enforcement (ICE) Detention Centers, 2020–2021

Emily C. Woods, MD, PhD, Jason R. Andrews, MD, and Jeremy D. Goldhaber-Fiebert, PhD

Objectives. To determine facility-level factors associated with COVID-19 outbreaks in US Immigration and Customs Enforcement (ICE) detention centers.

Methods. We obtained COVID-19 case counts at 88 ICE detention facilities from May 6, 2020, through June 21, 2021, from the COVID Prison Project. We obtained information about facility population size, facility type (dedicated to immigrants or mixed with other incarcerated populations), and facility operator (public vs private contractor) from third-party sources. We defined the threshold for a COVID-19 outbreak as a cumulative 3-week incidence of 10% or more of the detained population.

Results. Sixty-three facilities (72%) had at least 1 outbreak. Facilities with any outbreak were significantly more likely to be privately operated ($P < .001$), to have larger populations (113 vs 37; $P = .002$), and to have greater changes in their population size over the study period (–56% vs −26%; $P < .001$).

Conclusions. Several facility-level factors were associated with the occurrence of COVID-19 outbreaks in ICE facilities.

Public Health Implications. Structural and organizational factors that promote respiratory infection spread in ICE facilities must be addressed to protect detainee health. (*Am J Public Health*. 2024;114(9):909–912. https://doi.org/10.2105/AJPH.2024.307704)

AJPH September 2024, Vol. 114, No. 9

In a system that perpetuates structural racism, thousands of immigrants, many without criminal convictions, are incarcerated in Immigration and Customs Enforcement (ICE) detention facilities annually.[1–3] While detained, immigrants face conditions that can adversely affect their health, including increased risk of respiratory infections.[1,3] COVID-19 case rates among immigrants in ICE facilities were approximately 13 times higher than in the general US population.[3] Reasons for these higher rates are multifactorial, including crowded conditions, limited health care access, and insufficient testing.[3,4]

ICE facilities are heterogenous, differing in population size, whether run by public entities or private contractors, and whether immigrants are mixed with other incarcerated populations. Little is known about whether these differences contribute to unequal infectious risks across facilities. In this study, we examined whether facility-level factors were associated with COVID-19 outbreaks at ICE detention facilities.

METHODS

We obtained detainee COVID-19 case counts from 148 ICE facilities from the COVID Prison Project data set, containing data extracted from ICE's website from May 6, 2020, through June 21, 2021.[5] We obtained facilities' population sizes during the study period from the Transactional Records Clearinghouse.[6] We obtained data concerning the facility operator (whether public or private) and the type of facility (dedicated to immigrants or mixed with other populations) from the National Immigrant Justice Center.[7]

We based descriptive information about the facilities' contexts on their state, including political leaning (which party's candidate received a state's electoral college votes in the 2020 presidential election[8]), community COVID-19 vaccination rates (percentage of state population vaccinated by the end of the study period[9]), and when states included incarcerated people in COVID-19 vaccine roll-outs ("early" if included in phase 1 or "late" if included after phase 1 or not explicitly included[10]).

We excluded facilities if there was no information regarding detainee case counts (n = 4), total population size (n = 9), operator type (n = 42), or whether dedicated or mixed (n = 3), or if there were daily reported case counts larger than the reported total population size (n = 2; Figure A, available as a supplement to the online version of this article at https://www.ajph.org).

The primary outcome assessed was the occurrence of any outbreak. The threshold for an outbreak was defined as a cumulative 3-week incidence of 10% or more of the detained population.[11] We used a percentage rather than an absolute case number to account for the wide range of facility population sizes (1–1408). We selected 10% to capture events that were more likely to represent spread within the facility (rather than situations such as new admits who arrived infected but did not cause infection spread). Lastly, we used incidence over 3 weeks to capture a variation in infection dynamics (Figure B, available as a supplement to the online version of this article at https://www.ajph.org).

We used R version 4.2.2 (R Foundation for Statistical Computing, Vienna, Austria) to perform the analysis. We compared continuous variables with the Mann-Whitney-Wilcoxon test and categorical variables with the Fisher exact test. To account for 24 comparisons made, we used a sequentially rejective Bonferroni test (original $\alpha = 0.05$).

Reference data and code are available on Github at https://github.com/woodsec20/ICE-COVID-outbreaks.

RESULTS

Of the 148 facilities in the COVID Prison Project data set, 88 met criteria for inclusion. Overall, facilities were evenly split by political leaning (50% each), 67% were located in states that included incarcerated people in later vaccination stages, and 88% were located in states with a low percentage (≤ 60%) of adults vaccinated against COVID-19 by June 2021 (Table 1). The median facility population was 77 (interquartile range [IQR] = 23, 213). Sixty-four percent of facilities were publicly operated, and 20% of facilities only housed immigrants ("dedicated"). Three of the facilities were family residential centers.

Out of the 88 facilities, 63 (72%) had at least 1 outbreak during the study period, with outbreak occurrences roughly paralleling case counts in the United States (Figure C, available as a supplement to the online version of this article at https://www.ajph.org). Compared with facilities with no outbreak, facilities with outbreaks were more likely to be privately operated ($P < .001$), to have larger populations (113; IQR = 40, 347 vs 37; IQR = 15, 88; $P = .002$), and to have larger reductions in their population over the study period (–56%; IQR = −75, −35 vs −26%; IQR = −43, −20; $P < .001$; Table 1). Dedicated facilities were more likely to have an outbreak ($P < .001$).

Because both private operator and dedicated facility were strongly correlated with occurrence of any outbreak, we compared facility characteristics within these categories. All of the dedicated facilities were privately operated. Private facilities tended to have larger populations, so dedicated facilities, which were all privately operated, also tended to have larger populations (Table 1).

DISCUSSION

The majority of ICE detention facilities in this study experienced at least 1 COVID-19 outbreak, and outbreaks were significantly more likely to occur in facilities that were privately operated, were dedicated to immigrants, and had larger populations. These 3 factors are correlated, as all dedicated facilities were privately run, and private and dedicated facilities both tended to have larger populations.

The changes in population size over the course of the study are likely related to changes in ICE policies during this time. ICE issued guidance early in the pandemic to encourage facilities to reduce their population size, which was primarily accomplished by decreased apprehensions and arrests while continuing releases and deportations.[4]

Privately operated facilities may have a higher risk for outbreaks because ICE facilities run by private contractors have historically had less oversight of adherence to ICE protocols.[12] This trend likely continued during the pandemic, promoting infection spread if safety protocols were not consistently followed. Because all dedicated facilities in this study were privately operated, it was not possible to determine whether there may have been additional qualities of dedicated facilities that placed them at increased risk for outbreaks.

Limitations

This study had several limitations, most notably possible selection bias. Out of the more than 200 facilities that house

TABLE 1— Descriptive Characteristics of Immigration and Customs Enforcement Detention Facilities: United States, 2020–2021

	Total	Any Outbreak	No Outbreak	*P*	Public	Private	*P*	Dedicated[a]	Mixed[a]	*P*
No. of facilities	88	63	25	. . .	56	32	. . .	18	70	. . .
Context, no. (%)										
Facilities in Democratic-leaning states[b]	44 (50)	30 (48)	14 (56)	.63	29 (52)	15 (47)	.82	11 (61)	31 (44)	.43
Facilities in states with prisoners in late vaccination phase[c]	59 (67)	45 (71)	14 (56)	.21	33 (59)	26 (81)	.037	13 (72)	46 (66)	.78
Facilities in states with low percentage of adults vaccinated against COVID-19[d]	77 (88)	57 (90)	20 (80)	.28	48 (86)	29 (91)	.74	15 (83)	62 (89)	.69
Facility factors, no. (%)										
Facilities with public operator	56 (64)	32 (51)	24 (96)	< .001*	56 (100)	0 (0)	. . .	0 (0)	56 (80)	< .001*
Facilities dedicated to immigrant detainees only	18 (20)	18 (29)	0 (0)	< .001*	0 (0)	18 (56)	< .001*	18 (100)	0 (0)	. . .
Median facility population (IQR)	77 (23, 213)	113 (40, 347)	37 (15, 88)	.002*	48 (17, 96)	312 (113, 428)	< .001*	407 (321, 509)	65 (19, 126)	< .001*
Median percent change in facility population size (IQR)	−46 (−69, −28)	−56 (−75, −35)	−26 (−43, −20)	< .001*	−33 (−62, −21)	−58 (−72, −46)	.002*	−56 (−72, −43)	−42 (−68, −22)	.1

Note. IQR = interquartile range. Counts are shown with percentage of facilities in that category in parentheses and *P* value computed with the Fisher exact test. Medians are shown with IQRs (Q1, Q3) and *P* value computed with the Mann-Whitney-Wilcoxon test.

[a]Dedicated facilities are those in which only immigrants are detained, whereas mixed facilities are those in which both immigrants and other incarcerated populations are detained.

[b]Democratic-leaning states were defined as states where the Democratic party candidate won the electoral college votes in the 2020 presidential election.

[c]Late vaccination phase was defined as any phase after phase 1.

[d]Low percentage of adults vaccinated against COVID-19 was defined as less than 60% of the adult population in the state having received at least 1 vaccination against COVID-19 by June 21, 2021.

*Significant by a sequentially rejective Bonferroni test with $\alpha = 0.05$ and 24 comparisons made.

ICE detainees,[1] only 148 were available in the COVID Prison Project data set, biasing toward facilities that participated in COVID-19 case reporting. Of those 148, only 88 had adequate information available for inclusion in this study, predominately because of insufficient supporting information from third parties. Reanalysis with a subset of originally excluded facilities did not meaningfully alter the results (Table A, available as a supplement to the online version of this article at https://www.ajph.org). This analysis also did not reveal any substantial shifts in the facility characteristics, such as the state-based context factors that we examined (Table A), suggesting that these excluded facilities did not systematically differ from the included ones.

Many facilities only reported during a portion of the study period. With the exception of 1 facility, the lack of data was at the start of the study period (Figure D, available as a supplement to the online version of this article at https://www.ajph.org), likely reflecting delays in facilities starting to report data rather than selective withholding of data. Selection bias may have been introduced if facilities that were slower to adopt data-reporting policies also adopted pandemic safety measures more slowly. Moreover, dependence on third parties for supporting information about facilities may have introduced inaccuracies. Lastly, our outbreak definition may have missed small outbreaks. With these limitations, the scope of COVID-19 outbreaks in ICE facilities is likely larger than what was captured in this study.

Overall, our results add to the literature by highlighting that the risk of detained immigrants contracting COVID-19 was not equal across facilities, with those operated by private contractors and those only detaining immigrants having a higher risk of COVID-19 outbreaks. On the other hand, there was no association between outbreak risk and any of the state-based context factors we examined.

Public Health Implications

Improved data collection, reporting, and transparency by ICE facilities would help elucidate how these facility-level differences arose and inform interventions to mitigate risk.[13] Moreover, these results build upon numerous studies that highlight the adverse health outcomes for detained immigrants.[1,2] We therefore urge the adoption of policies that prioritize alternatives to detention, especially during times of infectious disease outbreaks. It is critical to protect immigrant health by addressing organizational factors that promote infection spread in these facilities, but until the underlying systemic racism that leads to the large number of detained immigrants is addressed, immigrant health will continue to be at risk. AJPH

ABOUT THE AUTHORS

Emily C. Woods is with the Department of Pathology, Stanford University School of Medicine, Stanford, CA. Jason R. Andrews is with the Department of Infectious Diseases, Stanford University School of Medicine. Jeremy D. Goldhaber-Fiebert is with the Department of Health Policy, Stanford University, Stanford, CA.

CORRESPONDENCE

Correspondence should be sent to Emily Woods, Stanford Department of Pathology, 300 Pasteur Drive, Lane Building L235, Stanford, CA 94305 (e-mail: emilywoods@stanford.edu). Reprints can be ordered at https://www.ajph.org by clicking the "Reprints" link.

PUBLICATION INFORMATION

Full Citation: Woods EC, Andrews JR, Goldhaber-Fiebert JD. Likelihood of COVID-19 outbreaks in US Immigration and Customs Enforcement (ICE) detention centers, 2020–2021. *Am J Public Health.* 2024;114(9):909–912.

Acceptance Date: April 17, 2024.

DOI: https://doi.org/10.2105/AJPH.2024.307704

CONTRIBUTORS

E. C. Woods contributed investigation, formal analysis, software, visualization, and writing (original draft, review, and editing). J. R. Andrews and J. D. Goldhaber-Fiebert contributed conceptualization, supervision, and writing (review and editing).

CONFLICTS OF INTEREST

The authors have no potential or actual conflicts of interest to disclose.

HUMAN PARTICIPANT PROTECTION

Human participants were not involved in this study. The original data source on which this study is based presented COVID-19 cases in aggregate with no identifying information.

REFERENCES

1. Saadi A, De Trinidad Young ME, Patler C, Estrada JL, Venters H. Understanding US immigration detention: reaffirming rights and addressing social-structural determinants of health. *Health Hum Rights.* 2020;22(1):187–197.
2. Diaz C, Nwadiuko J, Saadi A, Patler C. Advancing research to address the health impacts of structural racism in US immigration prisons. *Health Aff (Millwood).* 2023;42(10):1448–1455. https://doi.org/10.1377/hlthaff.2023.00479
3. Singer EK, Molyneux K, Kaur K, Kona N, Malave GS, Baranowski KA. The impact of immigration detention on the health of asylum seekers during the COVID-19 pandemic. *SSM Qual Res Health.* 2022;2:100072. https://doi.org/10.1016/j.ssmqr.2022.100072
4. Office of the Inspector General. ICE's management of COVID-19: lessons learned for future pandemics. Department of Homeland Security. September 7, 2021. Available at: https://www.oig.dhs.gov/sites/default/files/assets/2021-09/OIG-21-58-Sep21.pdf. Accessed March 30, 2023.
5. UNC Re-imagining Health and Justice Lab. COVID Prison Project. August 13, 2021. Available at: https://github.com/healthandjustice/covid-prison-project/tree/main/data. Accessed March 1, 2023.
6. Transactional Records Clearinghouse. Detention facilities average daily population. Syracuse University. Available at: https://trac.syr.edu/immigration/detentionstats/facilities.html. Accessed March 1, 2023.
7. National Immigrant Justice Center. ICE detention facilities as of November 2017. Available at: https://immigrantjustice.org/ice-detention-facilities-november-2017. Accessed March 1, 2023.
8. Woolley J, Peters G. Statistics: 2020. The American Presidency Project. UC Santa Barbara. 2021. Available at: https://www.presidency.ucsb.edu/statistics/elections/2020. Accessed March 6, 2023.
9. Centers for Disease Control and Prevention. COVID-19 vaccinations in the United States. COVID Data Tracker. 2023. Available at: https://covid.cdc.gov/covid-data-tracker. Accessed March 6, 2023.
10. Wang EA, Brinkley-Rubinstein L, Puglisi LB. The case for prioritizing COVID-19 vaccines in prisons and jails. *The Appeal.* February 22, 2021. Available at: https://theappeal.org/the-lab/report/covid-19-vaccines-in-prisons-and-jails. Accessed March 6, 2023.
11. Chin ET, Ryckman T, Prince L, et al. COVID-19 in the California State Prison System: an observational study of decarceration, ongoing risks, and risk factors. *J Gen Intern Med.* 2021;36(10):3096–3102. https://doi.org/10.1007/s11606-021-07022-x
12. US Government Accountability Office. Immigration detention: additional actions needed to strengthen management and oversight of facility costs and standards. October 2014. Available at: https://www.gao.gov/assets/gao-15-153.pdf. Accessed March 30, 2023.
13. Lo NC, Gonsalves GS. Outbreaks in US migrant detention centers—a vaccine-preventable cause of health inequity. *N Engl J Med.* 2023;389(8):679–681. https://doi.org/10.1056/NEJMp2304716

Postrelease Risk of Overdose and All-Cause Death Among Persons Released From Jail or Prison: Minnesota, March 2020–December 2021

Katherine Hill, MPH, Peter J. Bodurtha, MPP, Tyler N. A. Winkelman, MD, MSc, and Benjamin A. Howell, MD, MPH, MHS

See also Berk and Brinkley-Rubinstein, p. 852.

Objectives. To determine mortality risk among those recently released from a Minnesota jail or prison.

Methods. Using linked prison, jail, and death records, our retrospective cohort study followed 99 065 people who were released from Minnesota jails and prisons between March 1, 2020, and December 31, 2021. We explored differences between jail and prison exposures regarding mortality using standardized mortality ratios.

Results. Adjusting for age and gender, we estimated that the rate of overdose death for people released from jail was 15.5 times that of the Minnesota general population. Overdose death rates for people released from prison were even higher at 28.3 times the rate of the Minnesota general population.

Conclusions. Drug overdose was the leading cause of death for people reentering their communities from both jail and prison in Minnesota—with opioids being the leading cause of overdoses. Overdose death relative to the general population was double the estimates from earlier studies among people leaving prison. Providing seamless access to medications for opioid use disorder during and after incarceration is important to lower the risk of death following release. (*Am J Public Health*. 2024;114(9):913–922. https://doi.org/10.2105/AJPH.2024.307723)

At year-end 2021, approximately 1.2 million adults were currently incarcerated in prisons in the United States.[1] Ultimately, 95% of people incarcerated in state prisons will be released from incarceration and return to their communities.[2,3] This reentry process is difficult, as returning individuals face significant barriers and frayed social and familial bonds that increase their risk of morbidity and mortality. Specifically, a lack of housing, employment, health care, and other social services—from direct, legal, and socially sanctioned discrimination—negatively affects physical, mental, and substance-related health.[4,5]

Multiple US-based studies indicate that reentry after prison is an especially sensitive period for people who use drugs, with the first few weeks after release being the time of highest risk. A seminal Washington State retrospective cohort study from 1999 to 2003 found that the risk of death during the first 2 weeks after release among those formerly incarcerated in prison was 12.7 times that of state residents without a prison incarceration exposure.[6] Subsequent cohort studies have found overdose to be the leading cause of death after release from prison, indicating that drug use can be a risk factor for death during reentry.[7,8]

Yet, a research gap exists, as most of the current literature focuses on those recently released from prison and there are few studies on outcomes for people recently released from jail. These exposure differences are likely important, as prisons typically hold people if they are sentenced for more than a year, and releases are planned; alternatively, jails collectively hold a larger number of people but for short

AJPH September 2024, Vol. 114, No. 9

periods of time with often unpredictable releases. The few studies that examine postrelease mortality risk for those incarcerated in jails explore the impact of medications for opioid use disorder (MOUD) provision on subsequent overdose upon community reentry.[9,10] Furthermore, to our knowledge, no studies directly compare postrelease mortality between jail and prison populations in the same locality, and few disaggregate substance-specific causes of overdose. Understanding variation in risk of death by incarceration type (i.e., prisons or jails) is critical to appropriately develop interventions that address mortality after release.

Although some research has explored factors related to incarceration experiences (e.g., time spent incarcerated), there is poor understanding of how incarceration in jail versus prison affects the risk of fatal overdose upon community reentry.[11,12] Moreover, the majority of postrelease mortality research is from 2010 or earlier, predating the emergence of fentanyl (i.e., the third and fourth wave of the overdose crisis) and the COVID-19 pandemic.[13,14] Using data from Minnesota, we aimed to link prison, jail, and death records from March 1, 2020, through December 31, 2021, to estimate and compare postrelease all-cause and overdose-specific mortality among people leaving jail or prison.

METHODS

This retrospective cohort study consisted of 99 065 people who were released back into the community from Minnesota State Department of Corrections (hereafter referred to as "prison") or from Minnesota Regional, County and Local Correctional, Detention and Jail Facilities (hereafter referred to as "jail") between March 1, 2020, and December 31, 2021. We selected people for entry to the cohort if they experienced their release from either jail or prison during the study period. An individual's release date was based on their last release (from either jail or prison) during the study period. For instance, if someone was incarcerated in a Minnesota jail or prison multiple times during the study period, only data from their most recent release during the study period were recorded.

Sources of Data

We used data sets from 3 different sources: (1) the Minnesota Department of Corrections (DOC) state prison data and detention data, (2) the Minnesota Department of Health's Office of Vital Records, and (3) the US Census American Community Survey. The Minnesota data sets were restricted by time, from March 1, 2020, to December 31, 2021, to ensure temporal comparability.

We identified people released from a Minnesota prison in a data set provided by the Minnesota DOC. The prison data set specified the date of any status changes and the corresponding status (e.g., confinement, discharge). We included people released from prison in the cohort if their status changed to indicate they were released (i.e., no longer in prison) during the study period. This included statuses of intensive supervised release, standard supervised release, parole, conditional medical release—COVID-19 related or otherwise—absconding, or escaping. We identified people released from a Minnesota jail in a data set provided by the Minnesota DOC aggregated from licensed regional, county, and local facilities across the state. The jail data set included records of the start and end dates of one's jail hold. We included people released from jail in the cohort if they were released from jail detention during the study period and did not have a subsequent incarceration in either jail or prison. Both data sets included key demographic information on an incarcerated person's date of birth, gender, and race (i.e., no data on ethnicity was recorded). We did not include individuals who died, or likely died, while incarcerated (n = 8) in our analysis.

Data obtained from the Minnesota Department of Health's Office of Vital Records represented all recorded deaths in Minnesota during the study period. Extracted demographic data from this data set included the decedent's sex, age in years, date of birth, marital status, education, and race/ethnicity. We also extracted information about the decedent's death that was relevant to our study for analysis: date of death, cause of death (e.g., heart failure, sepsis), and *International Classification of Diseases* (*ICD*)-*10* codes (Geneva, Switzerland: World Health Organization; 1992). *ICD-10* ACME codes are diagnosis codes that identify the underlying cause of death and are input by medical examiners and health care providers. For our primary outcome of interest—overdose fatality—we used *ICD-10* codes indicating that the underlying cause of death was from an undetermined intent or accidental acute poisoning from substances other than alcohol to define a drug overdose death: X40–44 and Y10–14. We also classified other causes of death (e.g., COVID-19) with *ICD-10* codes.

We linked the prison release, jail release, and vital records data sets at the individual level using 1-way hashing based on first name, last name, and date of birth. We also used 1-way hashing to identify individuals across multiple jail facilities where there was no common identifier. More flexible methods (e.g., common identifiers, probabilistic matching) were unavailable for these data sources. Although hashing in this way likely resulted in a lower match rate than other methods, disparities are likely conservative.

The 2020 US Census American Community Survey provided 1-year data on Minnesota-specific state-level population average estimates to determine how many people were at risk for death in Minnesota in the reference population. We used these data to generate weighted estimates of population size as well as information on the population distribution in terms of gender, age, and race/ethnicity.

Statistical Analysis

We tabulated sample characteristics for people released from a Minnesota jail or prison from March 1, 2020, to December 31, 2021, using data from DOC. We tabulated the sample characteristics for the adult Minnesota general population for comparison using weighted population estimates from the 2020 American Community Survey. We used the χ^2 test for categorical variables and the *t* test for continuous variables to compare the overall distribution of sample characteristics for people released from jail or prison.

We tabulated the frequency and percentage of all-cause mortality and overdose-specific mortality for the Minnesota general population and for people released from jail or prison. We used the pairwise Fisher exact test—because of small sample sizes—to determine whether the proportion of data between the people released from jail or prison were different for categorical variables, whereas we used the *t* test for continuous variables.

We calculated overdose mortality rates per 100 000 person-years for both jail and prison releases as well as the Minnesota general population. To increase comparability across data sets, as the American Community Survey data provided estimates per year, we calculated a person-year as the amount of time each person was in the cohort, rounded up to the nearest year. Consequently, we did not adjust person-time at risk for time incarcerated or time following an individual's death. For instance, if an incarcerated person was released in March 2020 and died in April 2020, we recorded them as having contributed 1 year of person-time to the total person-time at risk. This conservative approach to measuring time at risk not only ensured that person-time calculations were comparable between data sets but also increased assurance that any resulting findings would be robust. We calculated mortality rates as the number of deaths over total at-risk years. We used indirect standardization to gender- and age-adjust overdose mortality among people released from jail or prison to the Minnesota age and gender distribution. We generated 95% confidence intervals (CIs), and we considered *P* values less than .05 significant. We performed all statistical analyses using SAS software version 9.4 for Windows (SAS Institute Inc., Cary, NC).

RESULTS

We included 99 065 people released from jail and prison in Minnesota in our cohort, for a total of 135 126 person-years. Table 1 provides sample characteristics of the people released from jail (n = 92 804) and people released from prison (n = 6261), as well as the Minnesota general population (n = 4 338 103). Both the population of those released from jail and those released from prison were younger (mean = 35.8 and 37.5 years, respectively) than the general population (mean = 48.2 years), and more likely to be male (people released from jail: n = 67 824, 73.2%; people released from prison: n = 5673, 90.6%; general population: n = 2 145 075, 49.4%) and Black or African American (people released from jail: n = 20 688, 22.3%; people released from prison: n = 1987, 31.7%; general population: n = 240 891, 5.6%). There were statistically significant differences between the population of people released from jail and the population of people released from prison in the distribution of age ($P < .001$), gender ($P < .001$), and race ($P < .001$).

All-Cause Mortality

We tabulated all-cause mortality across the Minnesota general population as well as people released from jail and prison (Table 2). Our data illustrate that the distribution of causes of death is categorically different for people released from jail and prison than for the general population, as well as all explored demographic variables (e.g., the general population is much older at death on average than are those released from incarceration). Overdose deaths represented the leading cause of death for both people released from jail and prison (35.9% and 33.1%, respectively), whereas the general population of Minnesota had a much smaller proportion experiencing this cause of death (1.7%). However, the frequency of overdose deaths was not significantly different between people released from jail and prison during the study

TABLE 1— Characteristics of People in Minnesota and People Released From Minnesota Carceral Facilities, Stratified by Jail and Prison Releasees: March 1, 2020–December 31, 2021

Sample Characteristics	General Population (n = 4 338 103), No. (%) or Mean ±SE	Jail Releasees (n = 92 804), No. (%) or Mean ±SD	Prison Releasees (n = 6 261), No. (%) or Mean ±SD	P^a
Age, continuous, y	48.2 ±0.1	35.8 ±12.1	37.5 ±10.6	< .001
Age group, y				< .001
18–24	476 486 (11.0)	17 870 (19.3)	505 (8.1)	
25–34	760 810 (17.5)	31 141 (33.6)	2 314 (37.0)	
35–44	756 784 (17.4)	23 266 (25.1)	2 023 (32.3)	
45–54	652 443 (15.0)	11 894 (12.8)	900 (14.4)	
55–64	748 734 (17.3)	6 998 (7.4)	414 (6.6)	
65–74	550 290 (12.7)	1 506 (1.6)	85 (1.4)	
≥ 75	392 556 (9.0)	229 (0.3)	20 (0.3)	
Gender[b]				< .001
Male	2 145 075 (49.4)	67 824 (73.2)	5 673 (90.6)	
Female	2 193 028 (50.6)	24 825 (26.8)	588 (9.4)	
Race/ethnicity[c]				< .001
American Indian or Alaska Native	33 041 (0.8)	5 812 (6.3)	660 (10.5)	
Black or African American	240 891 (5.6)	20 688 (22.3)	1 987 (31.7)	
White	3 515 181 (81.0)	58 924 (63.5)	3 430 (54.8)	
Asian or Pacific Islander	198 289 (4.6)	2 525 (2.7)	166 (2.7)	
Unknown	. . .	4 855 (5.2)	18 (0.3)	
Hispanic	121 110 (2.8)	. . .	. . .	
≥ 2 races	214 894 (5.0)	. . .	. . .	
Other	14 697 (0.3)	. . .	. . .	

Note. Releases represent the most recent, last release for all individuals (i.e., each person is only represented once even if they were imprisoned and released multiples times in this period). The Minnesota general population represents weighted population estimates from the 2020 American Community Survey for those 18 years and older.
[a] *P* value is for the χ^2 test for categorical variables and the *t* test is for continuous variables, comparing the population of jail releasees and prison releasees.
[b] 155 missing observations from those who were incarcerated.
[c] The race/ethnicity categories differ between data sources. The prison/jail data sets only include American Indian or Alaska Native, Black or African American, White, and Asian or Pacific Islander. No information on Hispanic ethnicity is collected.

period ($P = .55$), although this comparison may not be adequately powered to detect a difference should it exist. Deceased people released from jail had a different distribution than did deceased people released from prison for specific age categories (25–34 years: $P = .01$; 55–64 years: $P = .01$; 65–74 years: $P = .04$; ≥ 75 years: $P = .01$), gender ($P < .001$), specific race/ethnicity categories (non-Hispanic Black or African American: $P = .004$; non-Hispanic White: $P = .025$), and education (eighth grade or less: $P = .027$; bachelor's degree: $P = .001$).

Overdose Fatalities

Table 3 provides information on the fatal overdoses among the Minnesota general population (n = 1605) and those released from jail (n = 360) and prison (n = 41). Opioid-involved overdose deaths were the leading cause of overdose fatalities, comprising more than 50% of all overdose deaths, regardless of subpopulation. There were high frequencies of fatal overdoses from combination opioid and methamphetamine use among those who were released from jail and prison (18.1% and 14.6%, respectively), which were higher than were those of the general population (8.9%). Comparing the people released from jail who died from an overdose to the people released from prison who died from an overdose, there were only statistically significant differences between age

TABLE 2— All-Cause Deaths Stratified by the General Population, Jail Releasees, and Prison Releasees: Minnesota, March 1, 2020–December 31, 2021

Sample Characteristics	General Population[a] (n = 93 198), No. (%) or Mean ±SE	Jail Releasees (n = 1 004), No. (%) or Mean ±SD	Prison Releasees (n = 124), No. (%) or Mean ±SD	P[b]
Cause of death				
Cancer	18 753 (20.1)	26 (2.6)	12 (9.7)	< .001
Cardiovascular disease	15 385 (16.5)	61 (6.1)	11 (8.9)	.24
COVID-19	9 373 (10.1)	25 (2.5)	13 (10.5)	< .001
Liver disease	1 950 (2.1)	39 (3.9)	2 (1.6)	.31
Overdose	1 605 (1.7)	360 (35.9)	41 (33.1)	.55
Transport accident	903 (1.0)	55 (5.5)	6 (4.8)	> .99
Suicide	1 214 (1.3)	124 (12.4)	10 (8.1)	.31
Alcohol	95 (0.1)	1 (0.1)	1 (0.8)	.21
Homicide	37 (0.1)	8 (0.8)	1 (0.8)	> .99
Other	43 883 (47.1)	305 (30.4)	27 (21.8)	.048
Age at death, y				
Continuous	76.0 ±15.9	40.3 ±14.3	47.6 ±15.5	< .001
18–24	635 (0.7)	140 (13.9)	10 (8.1)	.07
25–34	1 591 (1.7)	281 (28.0)	21 (16.9)	.007
35–44	2 366 (2.5)	228 (22.7)	23 (18.6)	.31
45–54	4 291 (4.6)	155 (15.4)	24 (19.4)	.2
55–64	10 719 (11.5)	143 (14.2)	29 (23.4)	.012
65–74	17 462 (18.7)	49 (4.9)	12 (9.7)	.036
≥ 75	56 134 (60.2)	8 (0.8)	5 (4.0)	.01
Gender				< .001
Male	48 028 (51.5)	828 (82.5)	117 (94.4)	. . .
Female	45 170 (48.5)	176 (17.5)	7 (5.7)	. . .
Race/ethnicity[c]				
Non-Hispanic American Indian/Alaska Native	1 315 (1.4)	110 (11.0)	13 (10.7)	>.99
Non-Hispanic Black/African American	3 456 (3.7)	203 (20.3)	40 (32.8)	.004
Non-Hispanic White	84 193 (90.9)	596 (59.7)	59 (48.4)	.025
Hispanic	1 396 (1.5)	39 (3.9)	4 (3.3)	> .99
Non-Hispanic Asian or Pacific Islander	1 675 (1.8)	14 (1.4)	3 (2.5)	.42
≥ 2 races	430 (0.5)	30 (3.0)	3 (2.5)	> .99
Other	185 (0.2)	6 (0.6)	0 (0.0)	> .99
Marital status[d]				
Married	34 499 (37.1)	126 (12.6)	9 (7.4)	.11
Divorced	15 331 (16.5)	216 (21.6)	34 (27.9)	.09
Never married	12 085 (13.0)	626 (62.5)	72 (59.0)	.43
Separated	213 (0.2)	7 (0.7)	1 (0.8)	.61
Widowed	30 887 (33.2)	27 (2.7)	6 (4.9)	.16
Not obtainable	28 (0.0)	0 (0.0)	0 (0.0)	. . .
Education[e]				
≤ 8th grade	6 236 (6.8)	16 (1.6)	6 (4.9)	.027
9th–12th grade, no diploma	5 814 (6.3)	138 (13.9)	19 (15.6)	.68
High school graduate or general equivalency diploma	40 040 (43.4)	556 (55.9)	76 (62.5)	.25
Some college credit, no degree	12 044 (13.1)	149 (15.0)	13 (10.7)	.22

Continued

TABLE 2— Continued

Sample Characteristics	General Population[a] (n = 93 198), No. (%) or Mean ±SE	Jail Releasees (n = 1 004), No. (%) or Mean ±SD	Prison Releasees (n = 124), No. (%) or Mean ±SD	P^b
Associate degree	9 541 (10.3)	69 (6.9)	6 (4.9)	.57
Bachelor's degree	12 602 (13.7)	60 (6.0)	0 (0.0)	.001
Master's degree	4 345 (4.7)	6 (0.6)	2 (1.6)	.07
Doctorate degree	1 676 (1.8)	1 (0.1)	0 (0.0)	> .99

[a]Does not include the jail or prison releasees presented here.
[b]*P* value is for the pairwise Fisher exact test for categorical variables and the *t* test for continuous variables, comparing the population of jail releasees and prison releasees.
[c]548 unknown observations for MN population, 6 unknown observations for jail releasees, 2 unknown observations for prison releasees.
[d]55 unknown observations for MN population, 2 unknown observations for jail releasees, 2 unknown observations for prison releasees.
[e]900 unknown observations for MN population, 9 unknown observations for jail releasees, 2 unknown observations for prison releasees.

(mean = 36.1 and 41.9 years, respectively; *P* = .005) and those who were non-Hispanic Black or African American (*P* = .013) and non-Hispanic White (*P* = .046)—with a higher proportion of overdose fatalities being among non-Hispanic Black or African American individuals after release from prison than after release from jail.

Standardized Mortality Rates

For all-cause and overdose-specific fatalities, Table 4 shows both unadjusted and age- and gender-adjusted standardized mortality ratios for people released from jail and prison compared with the general population. For all-cause deaths, after engaging an age and gender adjustment, both people released from jail and prison had a higher standardized mortality rate (SMR) than did the Minnesota general population (jail: SMR = 1.42; 95% CI = 1.33, 1.51; prison: SMR = 2.05; 95% CI = 1.69, 2.41). As the crude mortality rate in the Minnesota general population was 1060.1 per 100 000 person-years, this translated to an age- and gender-adjusted mortality rate of 1505.3 per 100 000 person-years in the postjail release population and 2169.2 per 100 000 person-years in the postprison release population.

When solely examining overdose fatalities, after adjusting for age and gender, both people released from jail and prison also had a higher standardized mortality rate than did the Minnesota general population (jail: SMR = 15.51; 95% CI = 14.93, 17.11; prison: SMR = 28.34; 95% CI = 19.71, 37.09). As the crude mortality rate in the Minnesota general population was 18.2 per 100 000 person-years, this translated to an age- and gender-adjusted mortality rate of 283.3 per 100 000 person-years in the postjail release population and 517.6 per 100 000 person-years in the postprison release population.

DISCUSSION

In Minnesota the risk of death following release from carceral settings, whether jail or prison, is substantially higher than in the general population, although driven by different causes of death. For people released from both jail and prison in Minnesota, drug overdose was the leading cause of death from March 2020 to December 2021. People released from jail or prison who were reentering their community were 15.5 times and 28.3 times as likely, respectively, to die of an overdose compared with an age and gender matched general Minnesota population. It is notable that when standardized to the age and gender distribution of Minnesota, the risk of death because of overdose following release from prison is higher than is following release from jail over the same time. This is the first study, to our knowledge, to use contemporaneous jail and prison release data in a state to generate standardized mortality rates for both exposures. Further research is needed to understand what drives this apparent difference; does it reflect differences in the (1) underlying risk of people incarcerated in these facilities, (2) exposure to different carceral exposures (e.g., length, frequency), or (3) reentry processes?

We also found that both all-cause and overdose-specific mortality rates after release from jail and prison were higher than were estimates from similar, earlier studies of postrelease mortality. The seminal study on risk of death following release from prison conducted by Binswanger et al. using data from Washington State from 1999

TABLE 3— Overdose Fatalities Stratified by Jail and Prison Releasees: Minnesota, March 1, 2020–December 31, 2021

Sample Characteristics	General Population[a] (n = 1605), No. (%) or Mean ±SE	Jail Releasees (n = 360), No. (%) or Mean ±SD	Prison Releasees (n = 41), No. (%) or Mean ±SD	P^b
Overdose cause				
Opioid	872 (54.3)	210 (58.3)	23 (56.1)	.87
Methamphetamine	210 (13.1)	36 (10.0)	4 (9.8)	> .99
Opioid and methamphetamine	143 (8.9)	65 (18.1)	6 (14.6)	.67
Other	380 (23.7)	49 (13.6)	8 (19.5)	.34
Age at death, y				
Continuous	42.0 ±14.2	36.1 ±11.5	41.9 ±12.1	.005
18–24	170 (10.6)	58 (16.1)	3 (7.3)	.17
25–34	411 (25.6)	126 (35.0)	11 (26.8)	.39
35–44	356 (22.2)	92 (25.6)	9 (22.0)	.71
45–54	317 (19.8)	54 (15.0)	10 (24.4)	.12
55–64	269 (16.8)	27 (7.5)	7 (17.1)	.07
65–74	64 (4.0)	3 (0.8)	1 (2.4)	.35
≥ 75	18 (1.1)	0 (0.0)	0 (0.0)	. . .
Gender				.42
Male	1068 (66.5)	283 (78.6)	35 (85.4)	. . .
Female	537 (33.5)	77 (21.4)	6 (14.6)	. . .
Race/ethnicity[c]				
Non-Hispanic American Indian/Alaska Native	149 (9.4)	46 (12.9)	7 (17.1)	.47
Non-Hispanic Black/African American	277 (17.4)	82 (22.9)	17 (41.5)	.013
White	1004 (63.0)	203 (56.7)	16 (39.0)	.05
Hispanic	85 (5.3)	11 (3.1)	0 (0.0)	.61
Non-Hispanic Asian/Pacific Islander	19 (1.2)	1 (0.3)	0 (0.0)	> .99
≥ 2 races	55 (3.5)	12 (3.4)	1 (2.4)	> .99
Other	4 (0.3)	3 (0.8)	0 (0.0)	. . .
Marital status[d]				
Married	189 (11.8)	24 (6.7)	0 (0.0)	.16
Divorced	312 (19.5)	55 (15.4)	7 (17.1)	.82
Never married	1039 (64.8)	275 (76.4)	33 (80.5)	.7
Separated	15 (0.9)	2 (0.6)	1 (2.4)	.28
Widowed	48 (3.0)	4 (1.1)	0 (0.0)	> .99
Education[e]				
≤ 8th grade	29 (1.8)	2 (0.6)	2 (4.9)	.05
9th–12th grade, no diploma	213 (13.5)	65 (18.2)	5 (12.2)	.4
High school graduate or general equivalency diploma	798 (50.4)	204 (57.1)	26 (63.4)	.51
Some college credit, no degree	261 (16.5)	58 (16.3)	8 (19.5)	.66
Associate degree	141 (8.9)	20 (5.6)	0 (0.0)	.25
Bachelor's degree	120 (7.6)	7 (2.0)	0 (0.0)	> .99

Continued

TABLE 3— Continued

Sample Characteristics	General Population[a] (n = 1605), No. (%) or Mean ±SE	Jail Releasees (n = 360), No. (%) or Mean ±SD	Prison Releasees (n = 41), No. (%) or Mean ±SD	P^b
Master's degree	17 (1.1)	1 (0.3)	0 (0.0)	> .99
Doctorate degree	5 (0.3)	0 (0.0)	0 (0.0)	. . .

[a]Does not include formerly incarcerated people.
[b]*P* value is for the pairwise Fisher exact test for categorical variables and the *t* test for continuous variables, comparing the population of jail releasees and prison releases.
[c]12 unknown observations for MN general population, 2 unknown observations for jail releases.
[d]2 unknown observations for MN general population, 3 unknown observations for jail releases.
[e]21 unknown observations for MN general population, 3 unknown observations for jail releasees.

to 2003 found a postprison release mortality rate of 777 deaths per 100 000 person-years[6]; an update of that study, using data from 2014 to 2019 found a postprison mortality rate of 747 per 100 000 person-years.[15] In comparison, using data from 2020 to 2021 in Minnesota, we found a mortality rate of 795 and 1394 deaths per 100 000 person-years after release from jail and prison, respectively. Focusing on overdose mortality, the more recent Washington-based study found prison release overdose-related mortality to be 216 deaths per 100 000 person-years,[15] whereas we found overdose-related mortality to be 285 and 461 deaths per 100 000 person-years following release from jail and prison, respectively. Although underlying demographic distribution and risk factors are likely different between these 2 states, it is worth noting the dramatically higher risk of all-cause and overdose-related death in our postprison release population.

It is also possible that provision of MOUD during incarceration, reentry services, and community-based treatments varied between Washington and Minnesota at the time of each study, although we do not have this data for such a comparison. Instead, we hypothesize that our data reflect the evolving overdose crisis, which has seen a dramatic increase in overdose deaths in recent years because of fentanyl and psychostimulants. Although the rise in overdose deaths has been seen across

TABLE 4— Carceral Setting-Specific Standardized Mortality Ratios (SMRs), Indirectly Standardized to Minnesota General Population for All-Cause and Overdose Deaths (per 100 000 Person-Years): March 1, 2020–December 31, 2021

Adjustments	General Population, Reference Crude Rate	Jail Releasees		Prison Releasees	
		Standardized Rate Estimate	SMR (95% CI)	Standardized Rate Estimate	SMR (95% CI)
All-Cause Death					
Unadjusted	1060.1	795.0	0.75 (0.70, 0.80)	1393.6	1.31 (1.08, 1.55)
Age-adjusted	. . .	2126.3	2.01 (1.88, 2.13)	3622.9	3.42 (2.82, 4.02)
Gender-adjusted	. . .	559.3	0.53 (0.50, 0.56)	805.6	0.76 (0.63, 0.89)
Age- and gender-adjusted	. . .	1505.3	1.42 (1.33, 1.51)	2169.2	2.05 (1.69, 2.41)
Overdose Death					
Unadjusted	18.2	285.0	15.61 (14.00, 17.22)	460.8	25.28 (17.23, 32.43)
Age-adjusted	. . .	281.3	15.41 (13.82, 17.00)	476.8	26.16 (18.15, 34.16)
Gender-adjusted	. . .	331.4	18.15 (16.27, 20.02)	606.0	33.25 (23.07, 43.42)
Age- and gender-adjusted	. . .	283.3	15.51 (14.93, 17.11)	517.6	28.34 (19.71, 37.09)

Note. CI = confidence interval. Person-years were calculated for full year periods, and only those with all demographic information are included in the analysis.

different populations, our results suggest they may have a disproportionate impact on people reentering society from jail or prison.

Our results are also the first to our knowledge to reflect a period following the start of the COVID-19 pandemic, which led to large decreases in carceral populations and was associated with a national decrease in life expectancy. This finding highlights the need for more research on how postrelease mortality differs across contexts and over time.

Of note, we did not find differences between the distribution of most sample characteristics (i.e., overdose cause, age, gender, marital status, and education) between people released from jail and prison who died from a fatal overdose. However, there was a statistically significant difference between the population of people released from jail and prison for race and ethnicity: non-Hispanic Black or African American people died from fatal overdoses at a higher frequency after release from prison than after release from jail. Our study additionally showed that there was a high frequency of combination opioid and methamphetamine overdoses among those reentering the community after incarceration in either jail or prison.

Limitations

A few key study limitations should be noted. To start, many recently incarcerated people died within days of their release, but their person-time was rounded up to the nearest year to increase comparability between data sets, artificially inflating their person-time at risk. This conservative approach provides confidence that the findings of increased risk of fatal overdose among incarcerated persons compared with the general population are robust. Furthermore, this method does not account for variation in risk of death over time following release, which has been well documented as higher in the immediate postrelease period. Although our approach robustly compares risk of death to the general population, it generates postrelease mortality risk that will underestimate risk of death in the immediate postrelease period. Additionally, for all jail and prison releasees, we calculated person-time from their most recent release (so someone with multiple incarceration experiences during the study period only had their last release mark the start of person-time at risk). Although this may left-censor person-time at risk, rounding to the nearest year likely decreased any potential bias from such censoring.

Second, key variables were missing from our data sets that could have improved our study. First, we ascertained race and ethnicity data for the deceased from the Minnesota Department of Health's Office of Vital Records; although these are likely to be of high quality, there may be some individuals who had a race or ethnicity listed that would not match their self-report. Additionally, people who have been released from incarceration but survived through the study period did not have ethnicity documented in this data set. Therefore, the Minnesota DOC—as well as other US carceral settings—should collect ethnicity data for incarcerated people to help improve data quality for health equity research. Furthermore, whereas provision of MOUD across correctional facilities in Minnesota likely had an impact on postrelease mortality, we did not have access to medical records from correctional facilities for this study, so we could not assess prerelease use of MOUD and its potential impact on postrelease mortality.

Third, the generalizability of our results could be affected by (1) the study period (e.g., the first 2 years of the COVID-19 pandemic, which ushered in temporary decreases in the incarcerated population); and (2) the location of our study (e.g., our data focused on Minnesota exclusively). Thus, estimates of postrelease mortality may not be generalizable to other periods or other states. Future research should explore whether other states have similar patterns of inequities found here.

During the current era of mass incarceration in the United States, the high risk of death following release from jail or prison has been repeatedly documented. Our study, updating these estimates, demonstrates that the risk for being at risk of death following release from jail or prison remains significantly higher than among the general population and, if anything, has increased. Potential policy solutions to reduce this excess death can address social determinants of health (e.g., housing), increase access to MOUD for incarcerated people, and improve the process of reentry with a focus on connecting people to both health care and harm reduction services. Additional research is needed to assess the impact of increasing access to MOUD and transitional services on postrelease overdose and all-cause mortality, especially following federal guidance to expand access to MOUD in carceral settings and to encourage use of the 1115 waiver to expand health care for returning citizens.[16,17]

Public Health Implications

Returning citizens are at very high risk for fatal overdose. Release from incarceration is a clear, critical point of intervention for jails, prisons, public health institutions, and health care providers. Interventions designed to reduce excess deaths among people released from jail and prison may include (1) offering to start opioid agonist medications (buprenorphine or methadone) in carceral settings (2) ensuring continuity of care from carceral facilities to the community (especially for MOUD), (3) training and providing naloxone to all people who are released from incarceration, and (4) ensuring that people released from incarceration have adequate housing and employment opportunities to provide the means to support ongoing treatment. AJPH

ABOUT THE AUTHORS

Katherine Hill is with the Department of Epidemiology of Microbial Diseases, Yale School of Public Health, New Haven, CT. Peter J. Bodurtha and Tyler N. A. Winkelman are with the eHealth, Homelessness, and Criminal Justice Lab, Hennepin Healthcare Research Institute, Minneapolis, MN. Tyler N. A. Winkelman is also with the Department of Medicine, Hennepin Healthcare Research Institute. Benjamin A. Howell is with General Internal Medicine, SEICHE Center for Health and Justice, and Yale Program in Addiction Medicine, Yale School of Medicine, New Haven, CT.

CORRESPONDENCE

Correspondence should be sent to Katherine Hill, 60 College St, New Haven, CT 06510 (e-mail: k.hill@yale.edu). Reprints can be ordered at https://www.ajph.org by clicking the "Reprints" link.

PUBLICATION INFORMATION

Full Citation: Hill K, Bodurtha PJ, Winkelman TNA, Howell BA. Postrelease risk of overdose and all-cause death among persons released from jail or prison: Minnesota, March 2020–December 2021. *Am J Public Health*. 2024;114(9):913–922.

Acceptance Date: May 5, 2024.

DOI: https://doi.org/10.2105/AJPH.2024.307723

ORCID iDs:

Katherine Hill https://orcid.org/0000-0002-6515-8701

Peter J. Bodurtha https://orcid.org/0009-0009-8368-3399

Tyler N. A. Winkelman https://orcid.org/0000-0002-9581-5223

Benjamin A. Howell https://orcid.org/0000-0001-6938-8347

CONTRIBUTORS

K. Hill completed the analyses and led writing of the article. P. J. Bodurtha and T. N. A. Winkelman assisted with data access. B. A. Howell conceptualized and supervised the study. All authors contributed to the analytical plan, discussed the results, and contributed to the final article.

CONFLICTS OF INTEREST

The authors have no conflicts of interest to report.

HUMAN PARTICIPANT PROTECTION

Per guidance from the Yale institutional review board for research with this type of data, this research is determined to not meet criteria for research requiring review.

REFERENCES

1. Carson A. Prisoners in 2021: statistical tables. 2022. Available at: https://bjs.ojp.gov/sites/g/files/xyckuh236/files/media/document/p21st.pdf. Accessed June 11, 2024.
2. Minnesota Department of Corrections. Adult facilities. Available at: https://mn.gov/doc/facilities. Accessed June 3, 2023.
3. Hughes T, Wilson D. Reentry trends in the United States. 2004. Available at: https://bjs.ojp.gov/content/pub/pdf/reentry.pdf. Accessed June 11, 2024.
4. Western B. *Homeward: Life in the Year After Prison*. New York, NY: Russell Sage Foundation; 2018. https://doi.org/10.7758/9781610448710
5. Morenoff JD, Harding DJ. Incarceration, prisoner reentry, and communities. *Annu Rev Sociol*. 2014;40:411–429. https://doi.org/10.1146/annurev-soc-071811-145511
6. Binswanger IA, Stern MF, Deyo RA, et al. Release from prison—a high risk of death for former inmates. *N Engl J Med*. 2007;356(2):157–165. https://doi.org/10.1056/NEJMsa064115
7. Binswanger IA. Mortality after prison release: opioid overdose and other causes of death, risk factors, and time trends from 1999 to 2009. *Ann Intern Med*. 2013;159(9):592. https://doi.org/10.7326/0003-4819-159-9-201311050-00005
8. Ranapurwala SI, Figgatt MC, Remch M, et al. Opioid overdose deaths among formerly incarcerated persons and the general population: North Carolina, 2000–2018. *Am J Public Health*. 2022;112(2):300–303. https://doi.org/10.2105/AJPH.2021.306621
9. Friedmann PD, Dunn D, Michener P, et al. COVID-19 impact on opioid overdose after jail release in Massachusetts. *Drug Alcohol Depend Rep*. 2023;6:100141. https://doi.org/10.1016/j.dadr.2023.100141
10. Lim S, Cherian T, Katyal M, et al. Association between jail-based methadone or buprenorphine treatment for opioid use disorder and overdose mortality after release from New York City jails 2011–17. *Addiction*. 2023;118(3):459–467. https://doi.org/10.1111/add.16071
11. Krawczyk N, Schneider KE, Eisenberg MD, et al. Opioid overdose death following criminal justice involvement: linking statewide corrections and hospital databases to detect individuals at highest risk. *Drug Alcohol Depend*. 2020;213:107997. https://doi.org/10.1016/j.drugalcdep.2020.107997
12. Patterson EJ. The dose–response of time served in prison on mortality: New York State, 1989–2003. *Am J Public Health*. 2013;103(3):523–528. https://doi.org/10.2105/AJPH.2012.301148
13. Ciccarone D. The triple wave epidemic: supply and demand drivers of the US opioid overdose crisis. *Int J Drug Policy*. 2019;71:183–188. https://doi.org/10.1016/j.drugpo.2019.01.010
14. Ciccarone D. The rise of illicit fentanyls, stimulants and the fourth wave of the opioid overdose crisis. *Curr Opin Psychiatry*. 2021;34(4):344–350. https://doi.org/10.1097/YCO.0000000000000717
15. O'Connor AW, Sears JM, Fulton-Kehoe D. Overdose and substance-related mortality after release from prison in Washington State: 2014–2019. *Drug Alcohol Depend*. 2022;241:109655. https://doi.org/10.1016/j.drugalcdep.2022.109655
16. Centers for Medicare & Medicaid Services. HHS releases new guidance to encourage states to apply for new Medicaid reentry section 1115 demonstration opportunity to increase health care for people leaving carceral facilities. April 17, 2023. Available at: https://www.cms.gov/newsroom/press-releases/hhs-releases-new-guidance-encourage-states-apply-new-medicaid-reentry-section-1115-demonstration. Accessed March 4, 2024.
17. White House. White House ONDCP director Dr. Rahul Gupta and senior advisor to the president Tom Perez op-ed on expanding access to treatment for substance use disorder in correctional settings. January 29, 2024. Available at: https://www.whitehouse.gov/ondcp/briefing-room/2024/01/29/icymi-white-house-ondcp-director-dr-rahul-gupta-and-senior-advisor-to-the-president-tom-perez-op-ed-on-expanding-access-to-treatment-for-substance-use-disorder-in-correctional-settings. Accessed March 4, 2024.

Residential Proximity to Oil and Gas Development and Mental Health in a North American Preconception Cohort Study: 2013–2023

Mary D. Willis, PhD, MPH, Erin J. Campbell, BS, BA, Sophie Selbe, MPH, Martha R. Koenig, MPH, Jaimie L. Gradus, DSc, MPH, Yael I. Nillni, PhD, Joan A. Casey, PhD, MA, Nicole C. Deziel, PhD, MHS, Elizabeth E. Hatch, PhD, MS, Amelia K. Wesselink, PhD, MPH, and Lauren A. Wise, ScD, ScM

Objectives. To evaluate associations between oil and gas development (OGD) and mental health using cross-sectional data from a preconception cohort study, Pregnancy Study Online.

Methods. We analyzed baseline data from a prospective cohort of US and Canadian women aged 21 to 45 years who were attempting conception without fertility treatment (2013–2023). We developed residential proximity measures for active OGD during preconception, including distance from nearest site. At baseline, participants completed validated scales for perceived stress (10-item Perceived Stress Scale, PSS) and depressive symptoms (Major Depression Inventory, MDI) and reported psychotropic medication use. We used log-binomial regression and restricted cubic splines to estimate prevalence ratios (PRs) and 95% confidence intervals (CIs).

Results. Among 5725 participants across 37 states and provinces, residence at 2 km versus 20 to 50 km of active OGD was associated with moderate to high perceived stress (PSS ≥ 20 vs < 20: PR = 1.08; 95% CI = 0.98, 1.18), moderate to severe depressive symptoms (MDI ≥ 20 vs < 20: PR = 1.27; 95% CI = 1.11, 1.45), and psychotropic medication use (PR = 1.11; 95% CI = 0.97, 1.28).

Conclusions. Among North American pregnancy planners, closer proximity to OGD was associated with adverse preconception mental health symptomatology. (*Am J Public Health*. 2024;114(9):923–934. https://doi.org/10.2105/AJPH.2024.307730)

AJPH September 2024, Vol. 114, No. 9

An estimated 17.6 million US residents reside within 1 mile (1.6 km) of an active oil or gas development site,[1] and there is oil and gas activity close to many communities in Canada.[2] A wide range of geographies in both countries are affected by oil and gas development (OGD), although the amount of production varies by region based on geology (OGD production varies based on geology in, e.g., the key states CA, LA, OK, PA, and TX and the key provinces AB and BC).[2,3] This industry is projected to continue its rapid expansion in North America through 2050.[2,3] OGD produces air pollution, water contamination, and excess noise and light,[4–10] all of which may harm human health.[11–14] Previous work has identified associations between residential proximity to OGD and adverse health outcomes,[14] such as asthma exacerbations,[15–17] gestational hypertension,[18] preterm birth,[19–21] decreased birth weight,[22–24] and birth defects.[25,26]

Beyond their environmental hazards, extractive industries, such as OGD, create cycles of boom-and-bust economies, resulting in precarious employment and social disruption for affected communities.[27–29] Although OGD can generate considerable revenue,[30,31] the economic advantages accrue primarily to those who own mineral rights or work in the gas industry. These individuals often do not live near extraction sites.[31] Local communities—the people most exposed to the impacts of OGD—have little input on siting decisions in their communities or on amelioration of extraction-related exposures.[32,33] The confluence of swiftly changing economic, social, and environmental community conditions[34,35] may create stress and anxiety among residents who live nearby (Figure A, available as a supplement to the online version of this article at http://www.ajph.org).[27,31]

Previous work has documented that as OGD enters communities, there is an increased prevalence of psychological stressors[34,35] and symptoms of depression and anxiety.[36–40] This association is stronger among women and pregnant populations.[34,36–38] Although maternal mental health is a growing research area,[41] the preconception period remains understudied relative to the prenatal and postpartum periods.[42,43] Worse preconception mental health has been associated with reduced fecundability,[44,45] irregular menstrual cycles,[46] pregnancy complications,[47] and adverse birth outcomes.[47] Complex environmental, social, and economic exposures, such as those resulting from resource extraction, may be important risk factors for adverse preconception mental health.[48]

We investigated associations of residential proximity to and density of active oil or gas development with markers of psychosocial stress and depressive symptoms using baseline data from a North American preconception cohort study of couples trying to conceive without the use of fertility treatments.

METHODS

Pregnancy Study Online (PRESTO) is an ongoing Internet-based preconception cohort study of pregnancy planners who reside in the United States or Canada[49] and includes participants from every US state and Canadian province. Eligible participants were aged 21 to 45 years, identified as female, and were attempting to conceive without the use of fertility treatments. PRESTO recruited participants primarily through social media and health-related Web sites. After completing an eligibility screener questionnaire, participants completed a detailed baseline questionnaire on sociodemographic, behavioral, clinical, and reproductive factors. We used data from the baseline questionnaire and a cross-sectional study design.

Assessment of Exposure to Oil and Gas Development

We obtained data from a national database of OGD well locations in the United States and Canada: Enverus (formerly known as DrillingInfo, https://www.enverus.com). This database provides information on geographic locations of OGD (i.e., latitude and longitude coordinates), key dates (i.e., spud date, first production date, last production date, completion date), production type (e.g., oil, gas), and drilling type (e.g., horizontal, vertical, directional). Once a site was drilled, we considered the site active until it had an end date for production.

We assigned individual exposure metrics based on the proximity and density of active OGD sites within 20 km of the participant's address reported on their baseline questionnaire (Figure B, available as a supplement to the online version of this article at http://www.ajph.org). Using the date of their completed questionnaire, we also considered different time windows when calculating these metrics. We based metrics on sites active at the time of baseline questionnaire completion and included (1) proximity, defined as distance to the nearest active oil or gas development site; (2) intensity of new OGD, defined as the inverse distance-squared weighted sum of newly drilled OGD sites in the 3 years preceding the baseline questionnaire; and (3) intensity of all oil or gas development, defined as the inverse distance-squared weighted sum of OGD sites. Inverse distance-squared weighting is the standard for measurement in this area of work because it upweights closer sites that are likely more relevant for health.[13,50] Per the existing literature, the 20-km distance measurement is considered relevant to health because of the transport of emitted chemicals and alterations in the landscape.[6,14,28]

Assessment of Mental Health Outcomes

On the baseline questionnaire, participants completed the 10-item version of the Perceived Stress Scale (PSS), a measure of how unpredictable, uncontrollable, and overwhelming individuals find their life circumstances. This measure is reliable for recent stress in the previous 4 to 8 weeks and is highly correlated with acute physical symptoms and health care utilization.[51,52] They also completed the Major Depression Inventory (MDI), a 12-item measure of reported depressive symptoms over the previous 2 weeks. MDI sensitivity is 0.86 to 0.92 and specificity is 0.82 to 0.86, compared with clinician-diagnosed major depression.[53–55] Participants also reported their current use of any psychotropic medications for anxiety, depression, or other indications, such as sleep disorders (e.g., anxiolytics, anticonvulsants, antipsychotics, atypical antidepressants, benzodiazepines, beta-blockers, mood stabilizers, sedative hypnotics, selective serotonin-norepinephrine reuptake inhibitors, selective serotonin reuptake inhibitors, stimulants, tetracyclic antidepressants, tricyclic antidepressants).

Between June 2013 and July 2023, 17 356 eligible self-identified female participants completed the baseline questionnaire. We excluded participants if they did not complete the baseline questionnaire within 60 days of the eligibility screener (n = 47; 0.3%), provided implausible or missing data on last menstrual period date (n = 217; 1.3%), had more than 6 cycles of pregnancy attempts at time of enrollment (i.e., subfertility, a risk factor for stress and depressive symptoms; n = 3386; 19.5%), had a baseline residential address that could not be geocoded to the street level (n = 1321; 7.6%), or was greater than 50 km from 1 or more active oil or gas development sites (n = 6660; 38.4%). These criteria yielded 5725 participants for analysis.

Statistical Analysis

We examined sociodemographic characteristics of the cohort by exposure. Because of a lack of established clinical cutpoints for the PSS, we dichotomized scores based on distributions in the cohort: less than 20 (no to moderate stress) and 20 or more (moderate to high stress).[45] For MDI, we dichotomized scores following standard categories of depression symptomatology: less than 20 (no to low depressive symptoms) and 20 or more (moderate to severe depressive symptoms).[44,46,55] We dichotomized variables for psychotropic medication use (current vs none). We imputed missing covariate and outcome information (< 5%) using fully conditional specification methods, whereby we generated 20 data sets and statistically combined the standardized parameter estimates and SEs.[56]

For the proximity analysis, we generated restricted cubic splines to explore the nonlinearity in the association between residential proximity to OGD and each outcome variable. For the intensity analyses, we grouped participants into tertiles based on the density of sites (i.e., low, medium, or high), provided the participants resided within 20 km of at least 1 active site. In both the proximity and intensity models, the unexposed comparison group comprised participants living 20 to 50 km from OGD.

We used log-binomial regression models to estimate prevalence ratios (PRs) and 95% confidence intervals (CIs) for each mental health outcome variable. We selected covariates using the existing literature and a directed acyclic graph (Figure C, available as a supplement to the online version of this article at http://www.ajph.org). OGD is a multifaceted exposure and has been associated with many predictors of mental health (e.g., household income, substance use, educational opportunities)[14,27,31]; therefore, many potential covariates are likely mediators of the exposure–outcome relation and should not be included in our models.[57]

Adjusted models included the following covariates: age (< 25, 25–29, 30–34, 35–39, ≥ 40 years); geographic region of residence (Northeast [NY, PA], South [AL, AR, FL, KY, LA, MD, MS, OK, TN, TX, VA, WV], Midwest [IN, IL, IA, KS, MI, MN, MO, NE, OH, SD], West [AK, AZ, CA, CO, NM, UT, WY], Canada [AB, BC, MB, SK]); season of baseline enrollment (winter [December, January, February], spring [March, April, May], summer [June, July, August], fall [September, October, November]); and year of baseline enrollment (between 2013 and 2023).

In accordance with modern statistical methods,[58,59] our approach to interpreting data was based on an evaluation of the magnitude, direction, and precision of the effect estimates, rather than binary significance testing (e.g., *P* values).

Sensitivity Analysis

Given that subfertility can deleteriously affect mental health,[60] to reduce the potential for selection bias and reverse causation bias, we repeated our primary analyses with only the participants who (1) had no history of infertility, and (2) had attempted to conceive for fewer than 3 menstrual cycles at the time of study entry. We also repeated primary analyses with only the participants who reported living at their current address for 1 year or more or provided the same zip code for their previous address, as longer-term residence may indicate inability to relocate or more accrual of adverse social and environmental exposures from OGD.[33,61] We also restricted our participants to those with a baseline household income less than $50 000, as those with fewer monetary resources may not have the ability to move away from OGD if desired.[31]

Statistical Software

We derived spatial exposure measures using R Statistical Software version 4.2.2 (R Foundation for Statistical Computing, Vienna, Austria) and conducted geocoding and statistical analyses using SAS version 9.4 (SAS Institute, Cary, NC). We generated restricted cubic splines using the %GLMCURV9 macro in SAS.[62]

RESULTS

The total sample consisted of 5725 participants residing within 50 km of active oil or gas development. The mean age at baseline was 30.0 years, and participants reported a mean of 2.1 cycles of pregnancy attempt at time of enrollment (Table 1). Participants residing closer to OGD were less likely to have a graduate school degree (e.g., 0 to < 5 km: 36.1%; 20 to < 50 km: 40.5%) and to report an annual household income of $150 000 or more (e.g., 0 to < 5 km: 16.9%; 20 to < 50 km: 21.4%). However, other characteristics were similar across distance groups, such as identifying as non-Hispanic White (e.g., 0 to < 5 km: 83.4%; 20 to 50 km: 83.6%) and living in an urban residential location (e.g., 0 to < 5 km: 97.3%; 20 to < 50 km: 97.2%). Residential locations spanned the United States and Canada and included areas with extensive OGD (Figure 1).

We observed the highest perceived stress among those living closest to an OGD site (Figure 2). For example, the PR at 2 km versus 20 to 50 km was 1.08 (95% CI = 0.98, 1.18), and this association was attenuated at farther distances. The prevalence of moderate to high perceived stress was also greatest in the high category for the all-development intensity exposure metric (PR = 1.09; 95% CI = 0.99, 1.21) relative to the 20 to 50 km comparison group (Table 2).

For our continuous measure of distance to the nearest OGD site, we observed the highest prevalence of moderate to severe depressive symptoms out to 10 km, relative to the 20 to 50 km comparison group (Figure 2). The associations were most elevated between 0 and 10 km; for instance, the association at 2 km versus 20 to 50 km was 1.27 (95% CI = 1.11, 1.45). In the intensity models, we observed little evidence of an association between new OGD and depressive symptoms; however, the PR for moderate to severe depressive symptoms was elevated across the low and high, but not the medium, categories of the all-development intensity exposure metric (Table 2).

We observed a weak positive association between distance to nearest OGD site and current psychotropic medication use (Figure 2). For instance, the PR at 2 km versus 20 to 50 km was 1.11 (95% CI = 0.97, 1.28). We observed little evidence of an association for the all-development intensity exposure metrics, but the highest prevalence of current psychotropic medication use was among those living in the highest category of new development exposure intensity (PR = 1.27; 95% CI = 1.03, 1.55) relative to the 20 to 50 km comparison group (Table 2).

Results were similar, although less precise, among participants without a history of infertility (n = 5151) and participants with fewer than 3 cycles of pregnancy attempt at time at enrollment (n = 3741; Table A; Figure D [available as a supplement to the online version of this article at http://www.ajph.org]). We observed somewhat similar but less precise associations among those who resided in their home for 1 or more years (n = 3625) and among lower income participants (n = 1176; Table A; Figure D).

DISCUSSION

Using cross-sectional data from a North American preconception cohort study, we found a greater prevalence of adverse mental health outcomes among participants residing closer to more active OGD. Our study is among the first to examine associations of residential proximity to OGD across the United States and Canada and focused on a population that may be highly susceptible to the health risks associated with the industry.[14,27,31] Specifically, proximity to active OGD was associated with elevated levels of perceived stress and depressive symptoms. Intensity of active OGD was also associated with greater levels of depressive symptoms, whereas intensity of newly drilled OGD was associated with current psychotropic medication use only. These results provide support for the hypothesis that resource-extractive industries, such as OGD, pose a hazard for the mental health of local communities.

Health-protective policies related to OGD often focus on setback distances (i.e., the minimum distance allowed between an oil or gas extraction site and a residential building) from sensitive receptors (e.g., homes, schools, health clinics).[63–65] The associations observed in our analyses persist farther away from the development sites than regulatory setback distances in most communities[63,65] Many states and provinces with extensive OGD activity, such as Colorado, Pennsylvania, and Texas, have had setback distances as small as 200 to 1000 feet (0.06–0.31 km).[63] California has proposed among the most stringent setback regulations in the United States, which would require 3200 feet (0.97 km) between new OGD and sensitive receptors.[66] Similar measures related to setback distances are being implemented in Canada, in Alberta, Manitoba, and Saskatchewan.[67–69] We found associations between OGD and adverse mental health out to 2 km, even as far away as 18 km for depressive symptoms. Our results generally align with a recent expert consensus on

TABLE 1— Baseline Characteristics of Participants by Residential Proximity to Oil and Gas Development: Pregnancy Study Online, United States and Canada, 2013–2023

Characteristic	All Participants	Distance From the Nearest Active Oil or Gas Development Site, km				
		0 to < 5	5 to < 10	10 to < 15	15 to < 20	20 to < 50
Total participants, no.	5725	1695	1055	678	613	1684
Mean age at enrollment, y	30.0	29.7	30.1	30.0	30.1	30.2
Mean pregnancy attempt time, cycles	2.1	2.1	2.0	2.1	2.0	2.1
Married to partner, %	88.2	87.6	86.7	88.9	89.9	88.5
Race/ethnicity, %[a]						
Non-Hispanic White	82.9	83.4	80.6	83.0	82.5	83.6
Non-Hispanic Black	3.4	3.7	4.0	2.4	2.5	3.5
Hispanic/Latina	7.2	6.5	7.7	8.2	7.7	7.0
Educational attainment, %						
< bachelor's degree	28.2	31.3	27.0	26.5	24.0	28.0
Bachelor's degree	33.5	32.5	37.5	36.0	35.6	31.4
Graduate school	38.4	36.1	37.3	37.5	40.4	40.5
Annual household income, US$, %						
< 50 000	20.5	21.1	20.9	19.3	20.2	20.5
50 000–99 999	36.3	38.4	36.2	34.4	34.3	35.6
100 000–149 999	24.3	23.6	26.3	26.8	25.1	22.4
≥ 150 000	18.8	16.9	16.6	19.5	20.5	21.4
Current smoker, %	6.2	7.9	7.0	4.6	3.9	5.3
No primary care physician visits in the last year, %	13.0	13.0	12.5	10.4	10.9	14.8
Ever been pregnant, %	53.1	54.2	51.8	52.8	49.2	53.7
History of infertility, %	10.0	11.4	9.9	9.1	8.0	9.7
Season of baseline enrollment, %						
Winter	28.4	28.5	26.0	30.7	25.1	29.7
Spring	24.9	24.3	25.0	21.2	27.3	26.1
Summer	23.9	24.0	25.8	24.5	23.8	22.6
Fall	22.8	23.1	23.1	23.5	23.8	21.6
Physician-diagnosed medical conditions, %						
Anxiety	27.2	26.6	27.0	28.8	28.6	26.4
Depression	26.8	28.8	27.4	26.3	28.6	25.8
Diabetes	1.7	2.7	1.3	1.2	1.3	1.3
Endometriosis	3.5	3.5	3.8	4.0	2.6	3.6
Polycystic ovarian syndrome	10.0	9.4	9.6	8.1	9.1	10.5
Thyroid condition	7.4	7.9	5.6	6.9	7.3	7.7
Urbanized residential location,[b] %	97.2	97.3	97.2	97.2	97.2	97.2
Sleeps < 7 h/night, %	25.9	27.9	25.6	25.2	25.6	24.1
Uses anxiety or depression medications, %	16.4	17.5	16.9	15.9	13.7	16.2
Perceived Stress Score ≥ 20, %	30.2	32.0	29.0	29.0	27.4	30.3
Major Depressive Inventory score ≥ 20, %	18.4	19.9	19.4	19.4	15.1	15.7

Note. All participant characteristics were age-adjusted, except for age. Missing covariate and outcome information (< 5%) was imputed via a fully conditional specification method.

[a]Race/ethnicity data were derived via self-identification using categories, allowing participants to select all that apply, and conceptualized as a social and political construct.

[b]Urbanicity was defined differently by country using their respective census data. For the United States, we defined urban addresses as an area with a population density of at least 1000 people per square mile and with a population of at least 2500 people. For Canada, we defined urban addresses as in a census metropolitan area (an area consisting of ≥ 1 neighboring municipalities situated around an urban core with a total population of > 100 000 of which > 50 000 live in the urban core).

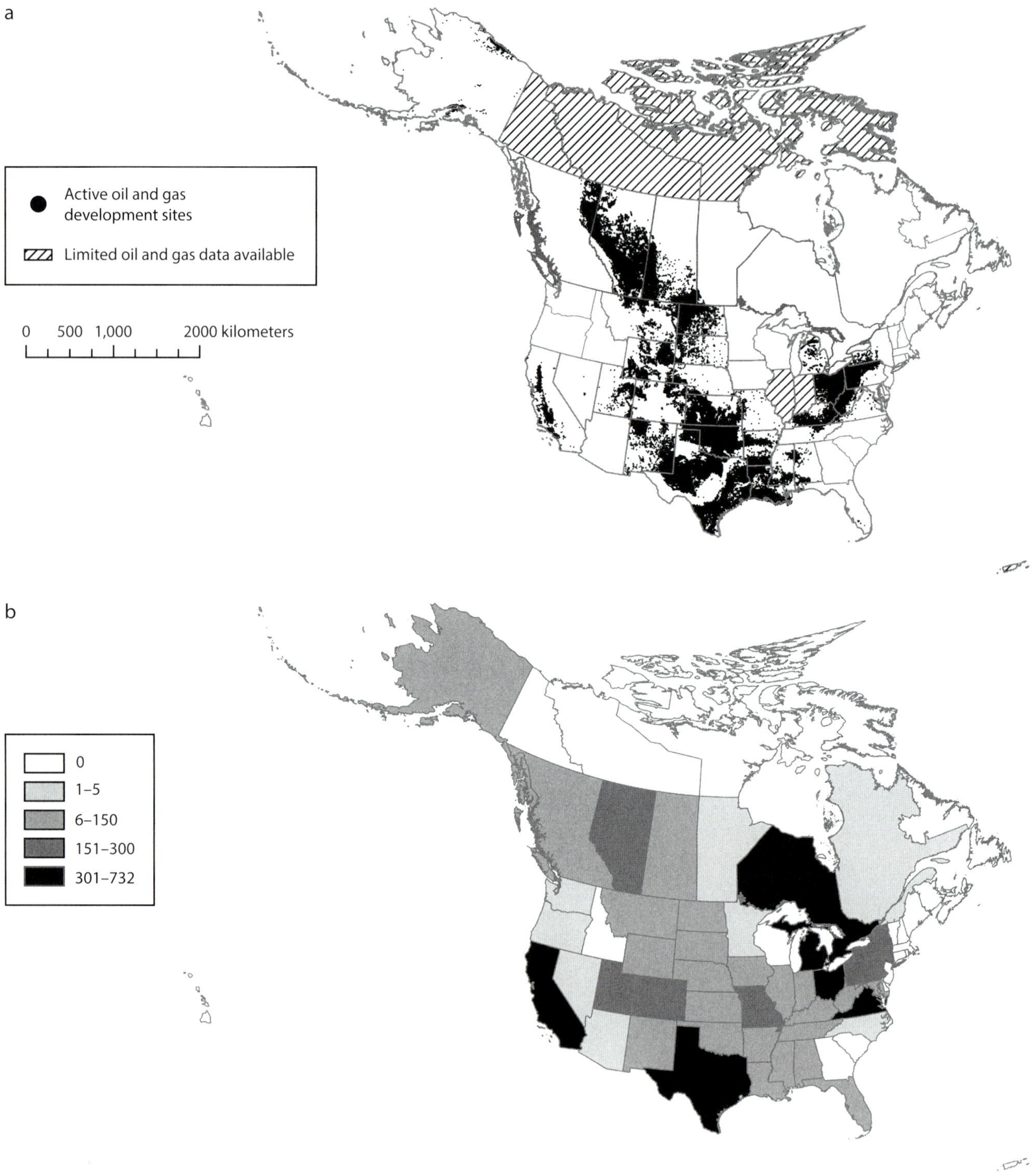

FIGURE 1— **Active Oil and Gas Development Sites by (a) Spatial Extent in 2022 and (b) Number of Participants Within 50 km of a Site: Pregnancy Study Online (PRESTO), United States and Canada, 2013–2023**

Note. A total of 1 151 504 active oil and gas sites were observed in the United States and Canada in 2022, and 5725 PRESTO participants resided within 50 km of an active oil or gas development site.

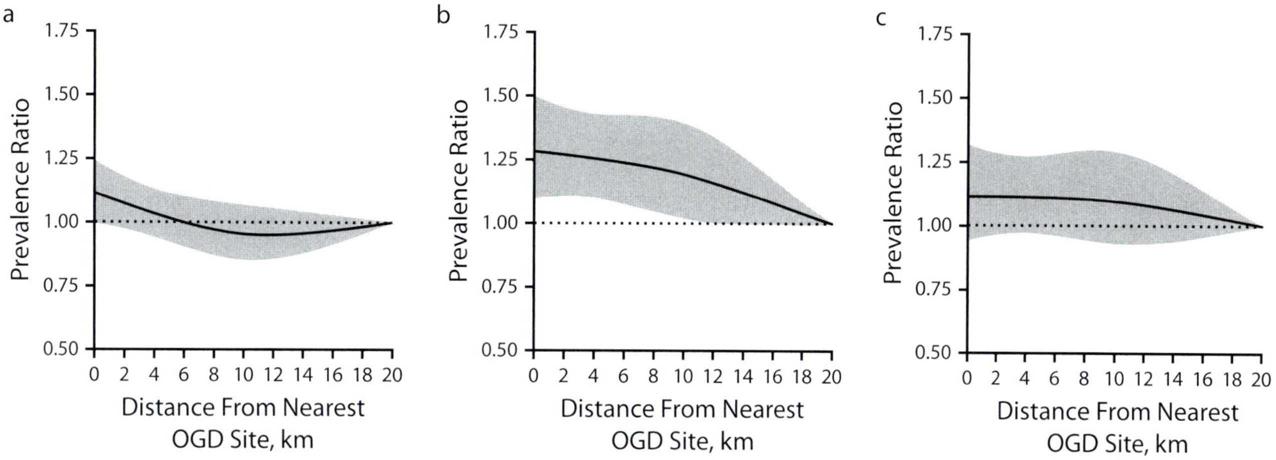

FIGURE 2— Associations Between Residential Proximity to Oil and Gas Development (OGD) Sites and (a) Perceived Stress Scale, (b) Major Depression Inventory, and (C) Current Psychotropic Medication Use: Pregnancy Study Online, United States and Canada, 2013–2023

Note. Results were fitted using restricted cubic splines. Solid line denotes estimates from the restricted cubic spline with corresponding 95% confidence intervals in the shaded bands. Reference group contains participants who had no residential exposure within 20 km of their home (i.e., the participants resided between 20 and 50 km from the nearest OGD site). Adjusted for participant age, geographic region of residential location, season of baseline enrollment, and year of baseline enrollment. Data were trimmed at the 0.5th and 99.5th percentile distance from nearest OGD site. Knots were located at 2.5, 10.0, and 17.5 km. Moderate to high perceived stress defined as PSS-10 scores ≥ 20, and moderate to severe depressive symptoms defined as MDI scores ≥ 20.

appropriate minimum setback distances to protect health.[64] Many of the proposed setback distance zoning policies apply exclusively to new OGD,[70] leaving behind an extensive geographic scope of existing extraction sites that we included in this analysis (i.e., the all-development intensity metric).

Our study population is unique: pregnancy planners enrolled in an Internet-based cohort. To our knowledge, we are the first to focus on the preconception period for OGD, which is of high interest given the existing literature on adverse birth outcomes (there are 25 or more separate studies of perinatal health to date, all of which relied on administrative records).[13,18,20,22,23,25,36] Although understudied relative to the prenatal period, optimizing mental health during the preconception period can improve health outcomes during the perinatal and postpartum periods for pregnant individuals and their infants, respectively.[43] For instance, worse preconception symptoms related to stress, anxiety, and depression are associated with reduced fecundability,[44,45] irregular menstrual cycles,[46] pregnancy complications,[47] and adverse birth outcomes.[47] Given the strong link between maternal mental health and birth outcomes, our results may explain some of the associations seen in the literature on OGD and adverse birth outcomes. Understanding what environmental hazards may harm mental health in the preconception period is critical for determining future prevention programs and informing health-protective policy.

Our results enhance the existing epidemiologic literature focused on perinatal mental health. Two previous quantitative studies found that higher levels of exposure to OGD during pregnancy are associated with adverse mental health outcomes.[36,37] In the broader population, other work has found that the psychological toll of the oil and gas industry is often stronger among women than men.[34,38] Most epidemiological analyses rely on electronic health records and medication orders to ascertain mental health outcomes and therefore may not capture associations with subclinical endpoints. Conversely, in using validated psychometric instruments, our study builds on previous results by showing that the largest magnitude associations were present for depressive symptoms at levels that may not have led to documented clinical care. We observed associations with current psychotropic medication use for the metric for new development exposure but not the metric for older development or for proximity, differing with the existing literature to some degree. Building on previous work in more localized communities (e.g., northeastern PA,[36,38,40] northeastern BC[37]), we captured a wide range of OGD exposure scenarios, as our participants resided across the United States and Canada.

Our findings are supported by a substantial body of work on how resource

TABLE 2— Associations Between Intensity of OGD and Mental Health Outcomes: Pregnancy Study Online, United States and Canada, 2013–2023

Exposure Metric	Participants, No.	OGD Sites Within 20 km, Median (Range)	Moderate to High Perceived Stress[a]		Moderate to Severe Depressive Symptoms[b]		Current Psychotropic Medication Use[c]	
			Prevalence (%)	PR (95% CI)	Prevalence (%)	PR (95% CI)	Prevalence (%)	PR (95% CI)
All OGD intensity[d]								
Comparison[e]	1 684	0 (0–0)	29.9	1 (Ref)	15.5	1 (Ref)	16.3	1 (Ref)
Low	1 339	2 (1–19)	29.6	0.97 (0.87, 1.08)	18.2	1.16 (0.99, 1.37)	14.6	0.96 (0.81, 1.13)
Medium	1 330	35 (1–270)	28.3	0.91 (0.91, 1.02)	17.4	1.07 (0.91, 1.26)	17.4	1.09 (0.93, 1.27)
High	1 372	846 (1–12 949)	33.0	1.09 (0.99, 1.21)	21.7	1.36 (1.17, 1.58)	17.4	1.08 (0.92, 1.28)
New OGD intensity[f]								
Comparison[e]	1 684	0 (0–0)	29.9	1 (Ref)	15.5	1 (Ref)	16.3	1 (Ref)
Low	473	1 (1–7)	31.5	1.03 (0.89, 1.17)	19.7	1.08 (0.90, 1.31)	16.3	1.01 (0.81, 1.25)
Medium	472	8 (1–39)	30.7	0.99 (0.86, 1.15)	18.0	0.99 (0.81, 1.21)	16.3	1.05 (0.85, 1.30)
High	486	52 (1–1 648)	29.8	1.03 (0.89, 1.19)	18.7	1.04 (0.85, 1.26)	18.5	1.27 (1.03, 1.55)

Note. CI = confidence interval; OGD = oil and gas development; PR = prevalence ratio. Adjusted for participant age, geographic region of residential location, season of enrollment, and year of enrollment. Missing covariate and outcome information (< 5%) was multiply imputed using fully conditional specification methods.

[a]10-item Perceived Stress Scale scores ≥ 20.

[b]Major Depressive Inventory scores ≥ 20.

[c]Self-report of current psychotropic medication use.

[d]Inverse distance-squared weighted number of OGD sites within 20 km of the residential location that were currently active at the time of the baseline survey. Low corresponds to the first tertile of exposure, and high corresponds to the third tertile of exposure.

[e]Participants residing 20–50 km from the nearest active OGD site to the residential location.

[f]Inverse distance-squared weighted number of OGD sites within 20 km of the residential location that were drilled in the previous 3 years before the baseline survey. Low corresponds to the first tertile of exposure, and high corresponds to the third tertile of exposure.

extraction (e.g., oil, gas, coal, rare minerals) and other industrial activity influences local populations and societal constructs.[27,61,71,72] Increased psychiatric caseloads often coincide with the introduction of resource extraction in a community,[73] regardless of the specific industrialized resource. This trend may be attributable to distress from experiencing environmental degradation,[34] rapid shifts in community social hierarchies,[61,74] uncertainty in how emissions may influence their health,[61,75] or even inability to influence where this industrial activity occurs.[61,64] Relentless cycles of economic growth and decline (i.e., boom-and-bust phenomena), as is common with resource extraction, create stressful conditions that can adversely affect mental health.[27] Although there are some examples of excellent community resilience,[28] few widely adopted initiatives exist to help communities adapt to the cyclical nature of a resource-oriented economy.[75,76] With this literature in mind, we hypothesized that similar community-level mechanisms may explain the associations observed in our analysis.

Limitations

Although we used an industry-standard spatial database to derive residential exposure estimates,[77] detailed data were unavailable on the operational factors that vary over the life cycle of OGD that may influence exposures (e.g., construction, fracking, production, flaring).[78] We did, however, examine nearest distance to an active site (i.e., key policy information) and intensity of OGD sites nearby (i.e., closer to true exposure). We also acknowledge that this measure imperfectly considers abandoned and orphaned sites. Although the spatial database includes data on most regions with OGD (Figure 1), it lacks detailed exposure information in specific US states (e.g., IL, IN) and Canadian territories (e.g., NT, YT, NU). Therefore, we are likely underestimating exposures on the borders of these areas. Our exposure analysis relied on the residential address reported at baseline, a commonly used proxy in spatial epidemiology,[79] but this decision can introduce exposure misclassification by not accounting for individual time–activity patterns.[80] Results from pregnancy planners also may not generalize to the general reproductive-aged population, as pregnancy planners may differ fundamentally from nonplanners.[81] Furthermore, some participants reported higher socioeconomic status and per household income and education than the general populations of the United States or Canada,[82–85] and more than 80% of our study sample identified as non-Hispanic White.

Conclusions

This geographically diverse study of pregnancy planners revealed an association between residential proximity to OGD sites and adverse mental health symptoms, particularly for depressive symptoms. We conducted the first analysis of preconception exposures to OGD, which may have implications for reproductive, pregnancy, and postpartum health. Regardless of potential causality, these findings can facilitate planning for increased access to mental health services in areas where new fossil fuel extraction is likely to occur. Given that OGD persists across the United States and Canada, future research investigating the mental health implications of resource extraction, including longitudinal follow-up of exposed communities, is warranted. AJPH

ABOUT THE AUTHORS

Mary D. Willis, Erin J. Campbell, Sophie Selbe, Martha R. Koenig, Jaimie L. Gradus, Elizabeth Hatch, Amelia K. Wesselink, and Lauren A. Wise are with the Department of Epidemiology, Boston University School of Public Health, Boston, MA. Yael I. Nillni is with the Department of Psychiatry, Boston University Chobanian & Avedisian School of Medicine, Boston. Joan A. Casey is with the Department of Environmental Health and Occupational Health Sciences, School of Public Health, University of Washington, Seattle. Nicole C. Deziel is with the Department of Environmental Health Sciences, Yale School of Public Health, New Haven, CT.

CORRESPONDENCE

Correspondence should be sent to Mary D. Willis, 715 Albany St, Department of Epidemiology, Boston University School of Public Health, Boston, MA 02118 (e-mail: mwillis1@bu.edu). Reprints can be ordered at https://www.ajph.org by clicking the "Reprints" link.

PUBLICATION INFORMATION

Full Citation: Willis MD, Campbell EJ, Selbe S, et al. Residential proximity to oil and gas development and mental health in a North American preconception cohort study: 2013–2023. *Am J Public Health*. 2024;114(9):923–934.

Acceptance Date: May 17, 2024.

DOI: https://doi.org/10.2105/AJPH.2024.307730

ORCID iDs:

Mary D. Willis https://orcid.org/0000-0002-0247-7983

Martha R. Koenig https://orcid.org/0009-0006-8804-9475

CONTRIBUTORS

M. D. Willis and E. J. Campbell curated the data and performed the formal analyses. M. D. Willis, J. L. Gradus, Y. I. Nillni, J. A. Casey, N. C. Deziel, E. E. Hatch, A. K. Wesselink, and L. A. Wise designed the methodology. M. D. Willis, E. E. Hatch, A. K. Wesselink, and L. A. Wise conceptualized the study. M. D. Willis and L. A. Wise acquired funding, administered the project, and supervised the study. E. J. Campbell, S. Selbe, and M. R. Koenig executed data and analysis validation. All authors participated in writing the original draft, reviewed and edited the article, and have read and agreed to the published version of the article.

ACKNOWLEDGMENTS

This work was supported by the National Institutes of Health (NIH; grants DP5-OD033415, principal investigator: M. D. W.; R01-ES028923, multiple principal investigators: E. E. H., L. A. W.;

R01-HD086742, principal investigator: L. A. W.; R00-ES027023, principal investigator: J. A. C.).
We are grateful to Michael Bairos (Boston University) for developing and maintaining the Web-based infrastructure of the Pregnancy Study Online (PRESTO), Tanran Wang (Boston University) for managing the PRESTO data, and Andrea Kuriyama (Boston University) for general study support.

Note. The contents of this article are solely the responsibility of the authors and do not necessarily represent the official views of the NIH.

CONFLICTS OF INTEREST

PRESTO has received in-kind donations from Kindara.com and Swiss Precision Diagnostics for primary data collection. L. A. Wise is a consultant for AbbVie, Inc. and the Gates Foundation. None of the other authors have any conflicts of interest to report.

HUMAN PARTICIPANT PROTECTION

The Boston University Medical Campus institutional review board approved our study protocol.

REFERENCES

1. Czolowski E, Santoro R, Srebotnjak T, Shonkoff S. Toward consistent methodology to quantify populations in proximity to oil and gas development: a national spatial analysis and review. *Environ Health Perspect.* 2017;125(8):1–11. https://doi.org/10.1289/EHP1535
2. Canadian Centre for Energy Information. Energy fact book: 2023–2024. Available at: https://energy-information.canada.ca/sites/default/files/2023-10/energy-factbook-2023-2024.pdf. Accessed January 29, 2024.
3. US Energy Information Administration. Annual energy outlook 2023. March 23, 2023. Available at: https://www.eia.gov/outlooks/aeo/index.php. Accessed January 29, 2024.
4. Health Effects Institute. Human exposure to unconventional oil and gas development: a literature survey for research planning. 2019. Available at: https://www.heienergy.org/publication/human-exposure-unconventional-oil-and-gas-development-literature-survey-research. Accessed June 17, 2024.
5. Elliott EG, Ettinger AS, Leaderer BP, Bracken MB, Deziel NC. A systematic evaluation of chemicals in hydraulic-fracturing fluids and wastewater for reproductive and developmental toxicity. *J Expo Sci Environ Epidemiol.* 2017;27(1):90–99. https://doi.org/10.1038/jes.2015.81
6. Gonzalez DJX, Francis CK, Shaw GM, Cullen MR, Baiocchi M, Burke M. Upstream oil and gas production and ambient air pollution in California. *Sci Total Environ.* 2022;806(pt 1):150298. https://doi.org/10.1016/j.scitotenv.2021.150298
7. Li L, Blomberg AJ, Spengler JD, Coull BA, Schwartz JD, Koutrakis P. Unconventional oil and gas development and ambient particle radioactivity. *Nat Commun.* 2020;11(1):5002. https://doi.org/10.1038/s41467-020-18226-w
8. Boslett A, Hill E, Ma L, Zhang L. Rural light pollution from shale gas development and associated sleep and subjective well-being. *Resour Energy Econ.* 2021;64:101220. https://doi.org/10.1016/j.reseneeco.2021.101220
9. Allshouse WB, McKenzie LM, Barton K, Brindley S, Adgate JL. Community noise and air pollution exposure during the development of a multi-well oil and gas pad. *Environ Sci Technol.* 2019;53(12):7126–7135. https://doi.org/10.1021/acs.est.9b00052
10. Gorski I, Schwartz BS. Environmental health concerns from unconventional natural gas development. *Oxf Res Encycl Glob Public Health.* [Published online: February 25, 2019]. https://doi.org/10.1093/acrefore/9780190632366.013.44
11. Adgate JL, Goldstein BD, McKenzie LM. Potential public health hazards, exposures and health effects from unconventional natural gas development. *Environ Sci Technol.* 2014;48(15):8307–8320. https://doi.org/10.1021/es404621d
12. Korfmacher KS, Elam S, Gray KM, Haynes E, Hughes MH. Unconventional natural gas development and public health: toward a community-informed research agenda. *Rev Environ Health.* 2014;29(4):293–306. https://doi.org/10.1515/reveh-2014-0049
13. Deziel NC, Clark CJ, Casey JA, Bell ML, Plata DL, Saiers JE. Assessing exposure to unconventional oil and gas development: strengths, challenges, and implications for epidemiologic research. *Curr Environ Health Rep.* 2022;9(3):436–450. https://doi.org/10.1007/s40572-022-00358-4
14. Deziel NC, Brokovich E, Grotto I, et al. Unconventional oil and gas development and health outcomes: a scoping review of the epidemiological research. *Environ Res.* 2020;182:109124. https://doi.org/10.1016/j.envres.2020.109124
15. Rasmussen SG, Ogburn EL, McCormack M, et al. Association between unconventional natural gas development in the Marcellus shale and asthma exacerbations. *JAMA Intern Med.* 2016;176(9):1334–1343. https://doi.org/10.1001/jamainternmed.2016.2436
16. Willis MD, Jusko TA, Halterman JS, Hill EL. Unconventional natural gas development and pediatric asthma hospitalizations in Pennsylvania. *Environ Res.* 2018;166:402–408. https://doi.org/10.1016/j.envres.2018.06.022
17. Willis M, Hystad P, Denham A, Hill E. Natural gas development, flaring practices and paediatric asthma hospitalizations in Texas. *Int J Epidemiol.* 2021;49(6):1883–1896. https://doi.org/10.1093/ije/dyaa115
18. Willis MD, Hill EL, Kile ML, Carozza S, Hystad P. Associations between residential proximity to oil and gas extraction and hypertensive conditions during pregnancy: a difference-in-differences analysis in Texas, 1996–2009. *Int J Epidemiol.* 2022;51(2):525–536. https://doi.org/10.1093/ije/dyab246
19. Gonzalez DJX, Sherris AR, Yang W, et al. Oil and gas production and spontaneous preterm birth in the San Joaquin Valley, CA: a case-control study. *Environ Epidemiol.* 2020;4(4):e099. https://doi.org/10.1097/EE9.0000000000000099
20. Casey JA, Savitz DA, Rasmussen SG, et al. Unconventional natural gas development and birth outcomes in Pennsylvania, USA. *Epidemiology.* 2016;27(2):163–172. https://doi.org/10.1097/EDE.0000000000000387
21. Whitworth K, Marshall A, Symanski E. Drilling and production activity related to unconventional gas development and severity of preterm birth. *Environ Health Perspect.* 2018;126(3):037006. https://doi.org/10.1289/EHP2622
22. Willis M, Hill E, Kile M, Carozza S, Hystad P. Associations between residential proximity to oil and gas drilling and term birth weight and small for gestational age infants in Texas: a difference-in-differences analysis. *Environ Health Perspect.* 2021;129(7):077002. https://doi.org/10.1289/EHP7678
23. Tran K, Casey J, Cushing L, Morello-Frosch R. Residential proximity to oil and gas development and birth outcomes in California: a retrospective cohort study of 2006–2015 births. *Environ Health Perspect.* 2020;128(6):067001. https://doi.org/10.1289/EHP5842
24. Caron-Beaudoin É, Whitworth KW, Bosson-Rieutort D, Wendling G, Liu S, Verner MA. Density and proximity to hydraulic fracturing wells and birth outcomes in northeastern British Columbia, Canada. *J Expo Sci Environ Epidemiol.* 2021;31(1):53–61. https://doi.org/10.1038/s41370-020-0245-z
25. Willis MD, Carozza SE, Hystad P. Congenital anomalies associated with oil and gas development and resource extraction: a population-based retrospective cohort study in Texas. *J Expo Sci Environ Epidemiol.* 2023;33(1):84–93. https://doi.org/10.1038/s41370-022-00505-x
26. Gaughan C, Sorrentino KM, Liew Z, et al. Residential proximity to unconventional oil and gas development and birth defects in Ohio. *Environ Res.* 2023;229:115937. https://doi.org/10.1016/j.envres.2023.115937
27. Klasic M, Schomburg M, Arnold G, et al. A review of community impacts of boom–bust cycles in unconventional oil and gas development. *Energy Res Soc Sci.* 2022;93:102843. https://doi.org/10.1016/j.erss.2022.102843
28. Arnold G, Klasic M, Schomburg M, et al. Boom, bust, action! How communities can cope with boom–bust cycles in unconventional oil and gas development. *Rev Policy Res.* 2022;39(5):541–569. https://doi.org/10.1111/ropr.12490
29. Willis MD, Cushing LJ, Buonocore JJ, Deziel NC, Casey JA. It's electric! An environmental equity perspective on the lifecycle of our energy sources. *Environ Epidemiol.* 2023;7(2):e246. https://doi.org/10.1097/EE9.0000000000000246
30. Feyrer J, Mansur ET, Sacerdote B. Geographic dispersion of economic shocks: evidence from the fracking revolution. *Am Econ Rev.* 2017;107(4):1313–1334. https://doi.org/10.1257/aer.20151326
31. Black KJ, Boslett AJ, Hill EL, Ma L, McCoy SJ. Economic, environmental, and health impacts of the fracking boom. *Annu Rev Resour Econ.* 2021;13:311–334. https://doi.org/10.1146/annurev-resource-110320-092648
32. Kroepsch AC, Maniloff PT, Adgate JL, McKenzie LM, Dickinson KL. Environmental justice in unconventional oil and natural gas drilling and production: a critical review and research agenda. *Environ Sci Technol.* 2019;53(12):6601–6615. https://doi.org/10.1021/acs.est.9b00209
33. Malin SA. Depressed democracy, environmental injustice: exploring the negative mental health implications of unconventional oil and gas production in the United States. *Energy Res Soc Sci.* 2020;70:101720. https://doi.org/10.1016/j.erss.2020.101720
34. Elser H, Goldman-Mellor S, Morello-Frosch R, Deziel NC, Ranjbar K, Casey JA. Petro-riskscapes and environmental distress in West Texas: community perceptions of environmental

degradation, threats, and loss. *Energy Res Soc Sci.* 2020;
70:101798. https://doi.org/10.1016/j.erss.2020.101798

35. Hirsch JK, Bryant Smalley K, Selby-Nelson EM, et al. Psychosocial impact of fracking: a review of the literature on the mental health consequences of hydraulic fracturing. *Int J Ment Health Addict.* 2018;16(1):1–15. https://doi.org/10.1007/s11469-017-9792-5
36. Casey JA, Goin DE, Rudolph KE, et al. Unconventional natural gas development and adverse birth outcomes in Pennsylvania: the potential mediating role of antenatal anxiety and depression. *Environ Res.* 2019;177:108598. https://doi.org/10.1016/j.envres.2019.108598
37. Aker AM, Whitworth KW, Bosson-Rieutort D, et al. Proximity and density of unconventional natural gas wells and mental illness and substance use among pregnant individuals: an exploratory study in Canada. *Int J Hyg Environ Health.* 2022;242:113962. https://doi.org/10.1016/j.ijheh.2022.113962
38. Gorski-Steiner I, Bandeen-Roche K, Volk HE, O'Dell S, Schwartz BS. The association of unconventional natural gas development with diagnosis and treatment of internalizing disorders among adolescents in Pennsylvania using electronic health records. *Environ Res.* 2022;212:113167. https://doi.org/10.1016/j.envres.2022.113167
39. Soyer M, Kaminski K, Ziyanak S. Socio-Psychological impacts of hydraulic fracturing on community health and well-being. *Int J Environ Res Public Health.* 2020;17(4):1186. https://doi.org/10.3390/ijerph17041186
40. Casey JA, Wilcox HC, Hirsch AG, Pollak J, Schwartz BS. Associations of unconventional natural gas development with depression symptoms and disordered sleep in Pennsylvania. *Sci Rep.* 2018;8(1):11375. https://doi.org/10.1038/s41598-018-29747-2
41. Yeaton-Massey A, Herrero T. Recognizing maternal mental health disorders: beyond postpartum depression. *Curr Opin Obstet Gynecol.* 2019;31(2):116–119. https://doi.org/10.1097/GCO.0000000000000524
42. Harville EW, Mishra GD, Yeung E, et al. The Preconception Period analysis of Risks and Exposures Influencing health and Development (PrePARED) consortium. *Paediatr Perinat Epidemiol.* 2019;33(6):490–502. https://doi.org/10.1111/ppe.12592
43. Harper T, Kuohung W, Sayres L, Willis MD, Wise LA. Optimizing preconception care and interventions for improved population health. *Fertil Steril.* 2023;120(3 pt 1):438–448. https://doi.org/10.1016/j.fertnstert.2022.12.014
44. Nillni YI, Wesselink AK, Gradus JL, et al. Depression, anxiety, and psychotropic medication use and fecundability. *Am J Obstet Gynecol.* 2016;215(4):453.e1–453.e8. https://doi.org/10.1016/j.ajog.2016.04.022
45. Wesselink AK, Hatch EE, Rothman KJ, et al. Perceived stress and fecundability: a preconception cohort study of North American couples. *Am J Epidemiol.* 2018;187(12):2662–2671. https://doi.org/10.1093/aje/kwy186
46. Nillni YI, Wesselink AK, Hatch EE, et al. Mental health, psychotropic medication use, and menstrual cycle characteristics. *Clin Epidemiol.* 2018;10:1073–1082. https://doi.org/10.2147/CLEP.S152131
47. Witt WP, Wisk LE, Cheng ER, Hampton JM, Hagen EW. Preconception mental health predicts pregnancy complications and adverse birth outcomes: a national population-based study. *Matern Child Health J.* 2012;16(7):1525–1541. https://doi.org/10.1007/s10995-011-0916-4
48. Reuben A, Manczak EM, Cabrera LY, et al. The interplay of environmental exposures and mental health: setting an agenda. *Environ Health Perspect.* 2022;130(2):025001. https://doi.org/10.1289/EHP9889
49. Wise LA, Rothman KJ, Mikkelsen EM, et al. Design and conduct of an internet-based preconception cohort study in North America: Pregnancy Study Online (PRESTO). *Paediatr Perinat Epidemiol.* 2015;29(4):360–371. https://doi.org/10.1111/ppe.12201
50. Koehler K, Ellis JH, Casey JA, et al. Exposure assessment using secondary data sources in unconventional natural gas development and health studies. *Environ Sci Technol.* 2018;52(10):6061–6069. https://doi.org/10.1021/acs.est.8b00507
51. Cohen S, Kamarck T, Mermelstein R. A global measure of perceived stress. *J Health Soc Behav.* 1983;24(4):385–396. https://doi.org/10.2307/2136404
52. Lee EH. Review of the psychometric evidence of the perceived stress scale. *Asian Nurs Res.* 2012;6(4):121–127. https://doi.org/10.1016/j.anr.2012.08.004
53. Bech P. Quality of life instruments in depression. *Eur Psychiatry.* 1997;12(4):194–198. https://doi.org/10.1016/S0924-9338(97)89104-3
54. Bech P, Wermuth L. Applicability and validity of the Major Depression Inventory in patients with Parkinson's disease. *Nord J Psychiatry.* 1998;52(4):305–310. https://doi.org/10.1080/08039489850149741
55. Bech P, Rasmussen NA, Olsen LR, Noerholm V, Abildgaard W. The sensitivity and specificity of the Major Depression Inventory, using the present state examination as the index of diagnostic validity. *J Affect Disord.* 2001;66(2):159–164. https://doi.org/10.1016/S0165-0327(00)00309-8
56. Rubin DB. *Multiple Imputation for Nonresponse in Surveys.* Hoboken, NJ: Wiley; 2004.
57. Weng HY, Hsueh YH, Messam LLMV, Hertz-Picciotto I. Methods of covariate selection: directed acyclic graphs and the change-in-estimate procedure. *Am J Epidemiol.* 2009;169(10):1182–1190. https://doi.org/10.1093/aje/kwp035
58. Wasserstein RL, Lazar NA. The ASA statement on *p*-values: context, process, and purpose. *Am Stat.* 2016;70(2):129–133. https://doi.org/10.1080/00031305.2016.1154108
59. Savitz DA, Wise LA, Bond JC, et al. Responding to reviewers and editors about statistical significance testing. *Ann Intern Med.* 2024;177(3):385–386. https://doi.org/10.7326/M23-2430
60. Salih Joelsson L, Tydén T, Wanggren K, et al. Anxiety and depression symptoms among sub-fertile women, women pregnant after infertility treatment, and naturally pregnant women. *Eur Psychiatry.* 2017;45:212–219. https://doi.org/10.1016/j.eurpsy.2017.07.004
61. Malin SA, Ryder S, Lyra MG. Environmental justice and natural resource extraction: intersections of power, equity and access. *Environ Sociol.* 2019;5(2):109–116. https://doi.org/10.1080/23251042.2019.1608420
62. Li R, Hertzmark E, Spiegelman D. The SAS GLMCURV9 macro. September 10, 2008.
63. Haley M, McCawley M, Epstein AC, Arrington B, Bjerke EF. Adequacy of current state setbacks for directional high-volume hydraulic fracturing in the Marcellus, Barnett, and Niobrara shale plays. *Environ Health Perspect.* 2016;124(9):1323–1333. https://doi.org/10.1289/ehp.1510547
64. Lewis C, Greiner LH, Brown DR. Setback distances for unconventional oil and gas development: Delphi study results. *PLoS One.* 2018;13(8):e0202462. https://doi.org/10.1371/journal.pone.0202462
65. Fry M, Brannstrom C, Sakinejad M. Suburbanization and shale gas wells: patterns, planning perspectives, and reverse setback policies. *Landsc Urban Plan.* 2017;168(suppl C):9–21. https://doi.org/10.1016/j.landurbplan.2017.08.005
66. Governor Gavin Newsom. California moves to prevent new oil drilling near communities, expand health protections. 2021. Available at: https://www.gov.ca.gov/2021/10/21/california-moves-to-prevent-new-oil-drilling-near-communities-expand-health-protections-2. Accessed June 17, 2024.
67. Stevenson L. Well setback distances. February 13, 2023. Available at: https://www.manitoba.ca/iem/petroleum/infonotes/23-02.pdf. Accessed January 29, 2024.
68. Saskatchewan Association of Rural Municipalities. Oil and gas well setback distances. Available at: https://sarm.ca/associations/oil-and-gas-well-setback-distances. Accessed January 29, 2024.
69. Alberta Energy Regulator. Explaining AER setbacks. December 19, 2022. Available at: https://www.aer.ca/providing-information/news-and-resources/enerfaqs-and-fact-sheets/enerfaqs-setbacks. Accessed January 29, 2024.
70. Ericson SJ, Kaffine DT, Maniloff P. Costs of increasing oil and gas setbacks are initially modest but rise sharply. *Energy Policy.* 2020;146:111749. https://doi.org/10.1016/j.enpol.2020.111749
71. Peek MK, Cutchin MP, Freeman D, Stowe RP, Goodwin JS. Environmental hazards and stress: evidence from the Texas City Stress and Health Study. *J Epidemiol Community Health.* 2009;63(10):792–798. https://doi.org/10.1136/jech.2008.079806
72. Downey L, Van Willigen M. Environmental stressors: the mental health impacts of living near industrial activity. *J Health Soc Behav.* 2005;46(3):289–305. https://doi.org/10.1177/002214650504600306
73. Bacigalupi LM, Freudenberg WR. Increased mental health caseloads in an energy boomtown. *Adm Ment Health.* 1983;10(4):306–322. https://doi.org/10.1007/BF00823107
74. Sangaramoorthy T, Jamison AM, Boyle MD, et al. Place-based perceptions of the impacts of fracking along the Marcellus shale. *Soc Sci Med.* 2016;151:27–37. https://doi.org/10.1016/j.socscimed.2016.01.002
75. Jacquet JB. Review of risks to communities from shale energy development. *Environ Sci Technol.* 2014;48(15):8321–8333. https://doi.org/10.1021/es404647x
76. Weber JG. A decade of natural gas development: the makings of a resource curse? *Resour Energy Econ.* 2014;37:168–183. https://doi.org/10.1016/j.reseneeco.2013.11.013
77. Enverus. 2023. Available at: https://www.enverus.com. Accessed August 24, 2023.
78. US Department of Energy. Modern shale gas development in the United States: a primer.

April 2009. Available at: https://energy.gov/fe/downloads/modern-shale-gas-development-united-states-primer. Accessed January 19, 2018.

79. Elliott P, Wartenberg D. Spatial epidemiology: current approaches and future challenges. *Environ Health Perspect.* 2004;112(9):998–1006. https://doi.org/10.1289/ehp.6735

80. Healy MA, Gilliland JA. Quantifying the magnitude of environmental exposure misclassification when using imprecise address proxies in public health research. *Spat Spatiotemporal Epidemiol.* 2012;3(1):55–67. https://doi.org/10.1016/j.sste.2012.02.006

81. Cheng TS, Loy SL, Cheung YB, et al. Demographic characteristics, health behaviors before and during pregnancy, and pregnancy and birth outcomes in mothers with different pregnancy planning status. *Prev Sci Off J Soc Prev Res.* 2016;17(8):960–969. https://doi.org/10.1007/s11121-016-0694-8

82. Schrager NL, Wesselink AK, Wang TR, et al. Association of income and education with fecundability in a North American preconception cohort. *Ann Epidemiol.* 2020;50:41–47.e1. https://doi.org/10.1016/j.annepidem.2020.07.004

83. US Department of Commerce. Spotlight on US educational attainment. Available at: https://performance.commerce.gov/stories/s/U-S-Population-Spotlight-Educational-Attainment/na47-j74r. Accessed August 19, 2021.

84. Government of Canada, Statistics Canada. Canadian income survey, 2020. March 23, 2022. Available at: https://www150.statcan.gc.ca/n1/daily-quotidien/220323/dq220323a-eng.htm. Accessed February 22, 2023.

85. Government of Canada, Statistics Canada. Study: youth and education in Canada. October 4, 2021. Available at: https://www150.statcan.gc.ca/n1/daily-quotidien/211004/dq211004c-eng.htm. Accessed February 22, 2023.

Impact of Droughts on Served Drinking Water Disparities in California, 2007–2020

Sandy Sum, MA

Objectives. To quantify the impact of droughts on drinking water arsenic and nitrate levels provided by community water systems (CWSs) in California and to assess whether this effect varies across sociodemographic subgroups.

Methods. I integrated CWS characteristics, drought records, sociodemographic data, and regulatory drinking water samples (n = 83 317) from 2378 water systems serving 34.8 million residents from 2007 to 2020. I analyzed differential drought effects using fixed-effect regression analyses that cumulatively accounted for CWS-level trends, income, and agricultural measures.

Results. CWSs serving majority Latino/a communities show persistently higher and more variable drinking water nitrate levels. Drought increased nitrate concentrations in majority Latino/a communities, with the effect doubling for CWSs with more than 75% Latino/a populations served. Arsenic concentrations in surface sources also increased during drought for all groups. Differential effects are driven by very small (< 500) and privately owned systems.

Conclusions. Impending droughts driven by climate change may further increase drinking water disparities and arsenic threats. This underscores the critical need to address existing inequities in climate resilience planning and grant making. (*Am J Public Health*. 2024;114(9):935–945. https://doi.org/10.2105/AJPH.2024.307758)

AJPH September 2024, Vol. 114, No. 9

A growing concern in the United States today is the unequal distribution of contaminant exposure in tap water provided by community water systems (CWSs), which collectively serve approximately 95% of the nation's residents. This importance is underscored by recent large grants for drinking water needs: the Biden–Harris administration's $6.5 billion funding initiative for water infrastructure upgrades and the Environmental Protection Agency's (EPA's) $50 million drinking water grant for disadvantaged and underserved communities. Although environmental justice studies have documented unequal exposure to drinking water contaminants in the United States, there is limited understanding of how these disparities have evolved. Furthermore, smaller and resource-poor CWSs, often associated with such disparities, are likely to be more vulnerable to climate hazards. Droughts, in particular, have been identified as critical threats to water systems' ability to provide clean drinking water.[1] Despite the expected intensification of drought conditions,[2] few studies have examined how drought affects drinking water quality and whether its consequences vary across sociodemographic subgroups.

A rich literature has documented disparities in drinking water quality and explored their origins and persistence.[3–6] Balaz and Ray describe how a combination of natural, built, and sociopolitical factors collectively influence exposure to drinking water contaminants.[7] Consequently, disparities in drinking water often reflect broader inequalities in geographic locations, public infrastructure, and sociopolitical and financial resources. Low-income and minority communities often bear the compounding burdens of elevated contaminant exposure and inadequate water treatment infrastructure.[1]

Regional and nationwide studies have consistently documented that Latino/a communities are exposed to higher drinking water nitrate (DWN) concentrations.[3,5,6] A nationwide study found that CWSs with high nitrate levels (> 5 mg/l) served twice as many Latino/a residents as did low nitrate CWSs (< 5 mg/l).[5] CWSs that rely on groundwater, serving smaller populations, and serving Latino/a communities were associated with elevated arsenic concentrations.[4,6,8]

Arsenic and nitrate are widespread contaminants frequently found exceeding their respective legal limits.[9] Long-term exposure to arsenic and nitrate has been associated with various types of cancers and thyroid, skin, and cardiovascular diseases in adults and with developmental impairments and adverse birth outcomes for infants.[10–12] Both of these contaminants are colorless, odorless, and expensive to treat, posing challenges for detection and treatment.

I have added, to my knowledge, a novel dimension to the environmental justice literature on drinking water with my analysis of how past droughts have affected drinking water quality provided by California CWSs; this new dimension accounts for existing disparities. Drought conditions lead to large-scale changes in the sources of drinking water (e.g., rivers, reservoirs, and aquifers) that can affect arsenic and nitrate concentrations. These changes in water quality may or may not be passed on as drinking water to households, depending on the capability of the local CWS. The net effect of drought on contaminant concentration depends on the interaction between changes in water volume and local geochemical and hydrological factors.

A study in California's Central Valley found that drought conditions led to intensified groundwater pumping, which accelerated the downward migration of shallow contaminated water (the "downwelling" effect[13]), increasing nitrate levels in water supplies.[14] Studies indicate that drought-induced groundwater pumping can displace arsenic from clay sediments as land subsides[15] and that concurrent increasing nitrate concentrations may create geochemical conditions that lead to decreased arsenic concentrations.[16,17] Furthermore, high evaporation rates induced by elevated temperatures during drought conditions can concentrate contaminants in surface water and shallow groundwater.[18,19]

Both the federal government and the state of California have recognized the importance of providing safe drinking water for the public. Under the Safe Drinking Water Act (Pub L No. 93-523, 1974), the maximum contaminant levels (MCLs) for arsenic and nitrate in drinking water are 10 µg/l and 10 mg/l, respectively. In 2019, 64 and 48 CWSs in California violated the law by exceeding the MCLs for nitrate and arsenic, respectively.[20] The main sources of nitrate are runoffs from fertilizer and animal manure in agricultural regions, but they can also originate from sewage and septic systems in urban areas.[21]

California's long history of intensive agriculture has led to widespread nitrate pollution in water sources that are frequently used for drinking water supply.[14,21] Moreover, naturally occurring volcanic and granitic rocks in the state contribute to groundwater arsenic contamination.[18] As a result, drinking water issues arise, as not all CWSs possess adequate treatment capacity. A 2016 California Department of Water Resources report identified only 150 treatment facilities for nitrate and 79 for arsenic of 4463 water systems that serve permanent populations.[22] Importantly, these CWSs are not equally distributed across society, indicating that already vulnerable communities may be at heightened risk under climate change.

METHODS

I compiled a rich space- and time-varying data set of regulatory drinking water samples, sociodemographic characteristics of the populations served, historical drought records, measures of agricultural intensity, and CWSs' characteristics. Each record in the data set represents a contaminant concentration observed at a sampling point in the distribution system of a CWS for a specific year. I analyzed drought effects on drinking water arsenic (DWA) and DWN concentrations for the following CWS subgroups: all CWSs; nonmajority Latino/a CWSs; CWSs with more than a 25%, 50%, and 75% majority Latino/a population; and CWSs serving low-income and agricultural regions. I focused on contaminant levels instead of regulatory violations of the MCLs for 2 reasons.

First, emerging epidemiology studies have found adverse health and birth outcomes at exposure levels below the MCLs for both arsenic and nitrate.[10,23,24] People exposed to DWA at the MCL (10 µg/l) were 2.7 times (95% confidence interval [CI] = 1.2, 4.1) more likely to develop bladder cancer.[25] The nitrate MCL of 10 mg/l was set at the threshold associated with the onset of methemoglobinemia, an acute oxygen deprivation condition for infants, without consideration for any other long-term chronic exposure effects.[10] Recent epidemiological studies have found associations between nitrate concentrations below 5 mg/l and increased risks of colon cancer, thyroid cancer, and birth anomalies.[10,26] Increased nitrate exposures in the range of 0 to 6 mg/l were associated with elevated risks of limb and heart defects.[23]

Second, violation data are discretized, which masks persistent and informative changes in contaminant concentration levels below or above the MCLs. For instance, if drought triggers changes in nitrate concentrations below 10 mg/l, an analysis using violation data would fail to detect any effect.

Drinking Water Contaminant Data

I obtained nitrate and arsenic measurements from drinking water quality data for regulatory monitoring that was compiled by the California State Water Resources Control Board. Under the EPA standardized monitoring framework, CWSs are required to monitor and report nitrate concentrations at each entry point to the distribution system (sampling points) annually if previous nitrate concentrations were consistently low (< 5 mg/l) or quarterly if concentrations were higher. Arsenic monitoring is generally required once a year or every 3 years for surface and groundwater sampling points, respectively. Compliance rates are generally high: 4 (0.15%) and 37 (1.3%) of approximately 2800 CWSs serving residential populations in 2019 violated arsenic and nitrate monitoring requirements, respectively.[20]

CWSs can have multiple sampling points in the distribution system, which can be either ground or surface sourced and labeled "treated," "untreated," or "raw." To evaluate served drinking water quality, I employed a filtering method used in the drinking water literature.[4,27] This method filters out sampling points that are potentially upstream of a treatment plant, ensuring that measurements reflect the quality of served rather than source water. I assigned sampling points to each CWS-year, with the following prioritization: (1) treated sampling points and sampling points labeled as in the distribution system, (2) untreated sampling points, and (3) raw sampling points. For example, if (1) was available, I would drop (2) and (3). Raw sampling points remained in the study sample if they were the only sampling points associated with a CWS. Each CWS had an average of 3 sampling points representing served drinking water quality (Table 1).

For each remaining sampling point, I computed a time-weighted mean measure across observations in a given year for each contaminant. As in Pace et al., I replaced observations below the detection limit with zero.[6] I omitted sampling points with less than 4 observations for groundwater arsenic (required once every 3 years) and 8 observations for surface arsenic and both ground and surface nitrate (required annually) over 2007 to 2020. This criterion allowed the inclusion of CWSs that were unable to comply with EPA sampling requirements while providing sufficient observations for the identification of regression terms. I limited my main analysis to 2007 to 2020, starting a year after the EPA's 2006 Final Arsenic Rule, when CWSs were required to monitor for arsenic periodically.

Sociodemographic Characteristics

I obtained the water system service area boundaries verified in 2021 from the California State Water Resources Control Board Geographic Information System portal.[28] To assign sociodemographic composition to a CWS, I collected annual census tract–level variables from 2009 to 2020 from the American Community Survey (ACS) 5-year estimates. As the ACS estimates were first released in 2009, I used values from that year as a proxy for 2007 to 2008.

For each tract, I computed the percentage of residents identifying as Hispanic, non-Hispanic White, non-Hispanic Black, and non-Hispanic Asian, as well as the proportion of adults with less than a high school education and who do not speak English "very well." I used median household income directly in the following calculations. I refer to the set of tract-level computed percentages and direct estimates collectively as "measures" in the following section.

I used the area-weighted mean approach to aggregate tract-level measures to CWS service area boundaries. I identified all tracts that were wholly or partially in each CWSs' service area. I calculated the mean of all overlapping tracts' measures and weighted them by the overlapping area (Appendix A, Section 1.1, available as a supplement to the online version of this article at https://www.ajph.org). After obtaining CWS-year sociodemographic measures, I assigned to each CWS-year the following binary indicators: $1\{> P\%\ \mathit{Latino/a}\}$ if the percentage of Latino/a residents served was greater than $P \in \{25, 50, 75\}$, $1\{\mathit{majority\ Latino/a}\}$ if the percentage of Latino/a residents was greater than the percentage of any other racial or ethnic group, and $1\{\mathit{low\ income}\}$ if residents' mean income was less than $47 000. Specifically, a CWS serving a community that is 40% Latino/a could be considered "majority Latino/a" if each of the other ethnic/racial groups individually made up a smaller percentage. I based the low-income threshold of $47 000 on the median California state income limit for 2019.

TABLE 1— Summary Statistics of Community Water System (CWS) Features: California, 2007–2020

	All CWSs	Nonmajority Latino/a CWSs	Majority Latino/a CWSs
Aggregate statistics on CWSs in study sample[a]			
Number of CWSs	2378	1732	646
CWS owner type, no. (%)			
Local government	830 (35)	593 (34)	237 (37)
Private	1548 (65)	1139 (66)	409 (63)
System size of population served, no. (%)			
Very small	1463 (62)	1126 (65)	337 (52)
Medium-large	559 (24)	407 (23)	152 (24)
Very large	356 (15)	199 (11)	157 (24)
Total population served, in millions	34.8	17.7	17.1
Total no. of sampling points	6969	4682	2287
Sociodemographic, mean ±SD			
Population served	14 770 ±104 420	10 277 ±63 834	26 923 ±170 902
% Latino/a residents	32 ±23	20 ±11	64 ±16
% adults with <high school education	11 ±7	7 ±4	19 ±7
% adults that do not speak English very well	2.13 ±3.50	2.04 ±3.68	2.38 ±2.95
Household income, $	76 052 ±31 431	80 620 ±33 397	64 113 ±21 412
Land use, mean ±SD			
% cropland (in 1 mi^2 radius)	15 ±23	11 ±19	25 ±28
Located in overdraft groundwater basin	0.3 ±0.5	0.2 ±0.4	0.5 ±0.5
Depth to groundwater, ft	102 ±91	88 ±86	123 ±94
Water quality sampling points and drought exposure, mean ±SD			
Drought (normalized PDSI)	0.4 ±0.2	0.4 ±0.2	0.5 ±0.2
Nitrate, mg/l	1.9 ±2.5	1.5 ±1.9	3.0 ±3.3
Arsenic, μg/l	3.3 ±6.4	3.2 ±6.5	3.7 ±6.1
No. of sampling points	3.0 ±4.5	2.7 ±3.9	3.6 ±5.9
No. of sampling points from groundwater	3.4 ±5.2	3.1 ±4.5	4.1 ±6.8
No. of sampling points from surface water	0.4 ±1.4	0.4 ±1.2	0.5 ±1.8

Note. PDSI = Palmer Drought Severity Index. Majority Latino/a CWSs are characterized by serving a higher percentage of Latino/a population than any other racial or ethnic group. Aggregated key statistics for all CWSs included in the study sample: California, 2020. Mean ±SD of sociodemographic, land use, and CWS sampling points and drought variables: California, 2007–2020. Because of observed differences in sociodemographic and land use variables between majority Latino/a and nonmajority Latino/a CWSs, I included these variables as controls in robustness checks of the main regression specification estimating the effects of drought on drinking water nitrate and arsenic concentrations (Appendix A, Figure B, available as a supplement to the online version of this article at http://www.ajph.org).
[a]Values are sum of variables over CWSs included in study sample.

I also considered errors originating from the ACS data that may have invalidated my results. To account for these errors, I used the margin of error estimates associated with each ACS variable to compute a CI for each CWS-year computed measure. I reassigned sociodemographic indicators to each CWS-year using a more conservative threshold. The results and a discussion of this sensitivity analysis are available in Appendix A, Figure A and Section 3, respectively.

Drought Measure

To characterize drought, I used the Palmer Drought Severity Index (PDSI). This index uses meteorological data, including temperature and precipitation, to measure overall dryness conditions. I obtained gridded (0.05° × 0.05°) PDSI data at a 5-day interval from the University of Idaho Climatology Lab.[29]

To compute CWS-year means, I calculated the mean of PDSI values of all grid cells in the year that laid within a

2.5-mile radius of each CWS service area boundary centroid. I normalized the CWS-year–level PDSI so that its mean and SD were 1 and zero, respectively. To ease interpretation, I multiplied the normalized PDSI by −1 so that a positive value corresponded to drier than usual, and a negative number corresponded to wetter than usual. In this way, parameter estimates can be interpreted as the effect of a 1 SD increase in dryness. Figure 1 illustrates this normalized index over 1994 to 2020 across California (see also Appendix B, available as a supplement to the online version of this article at https://www.ajph.org).

Measures of Agricultural Activities

I also compiled CWS-year measures of groundwater levels, agricultural well intensity, and agricultural land use. I sourced all data from the California Department of Water Resources (described in Appendix A, Section 1.3). I created another CWS subgroup 1{*agricultural*}, indicating that the percentage of cropland was more than 25% within a 1-mile radius of the CWS. The 25% cropland criterion represents the threshold for the 85th percentile.

Estimating Drought Impacts

The regression specifications for estimating drought's effects on contaminant concentrations are expressed in Equations 1 and 2:

$$(1) \quad C_{iwt} = \beta D_{wt} + \delta_i + \tau_w t + \epsilon_{iwt}$$

$$(2) \quad C_{iwt} = \beta_0 D_{wt} + \beta_1 D_{wt} \times \mathbf{1}\{X\}_{wt} + \delta_i + \tau_w t + \epsilon_{iwt}$$

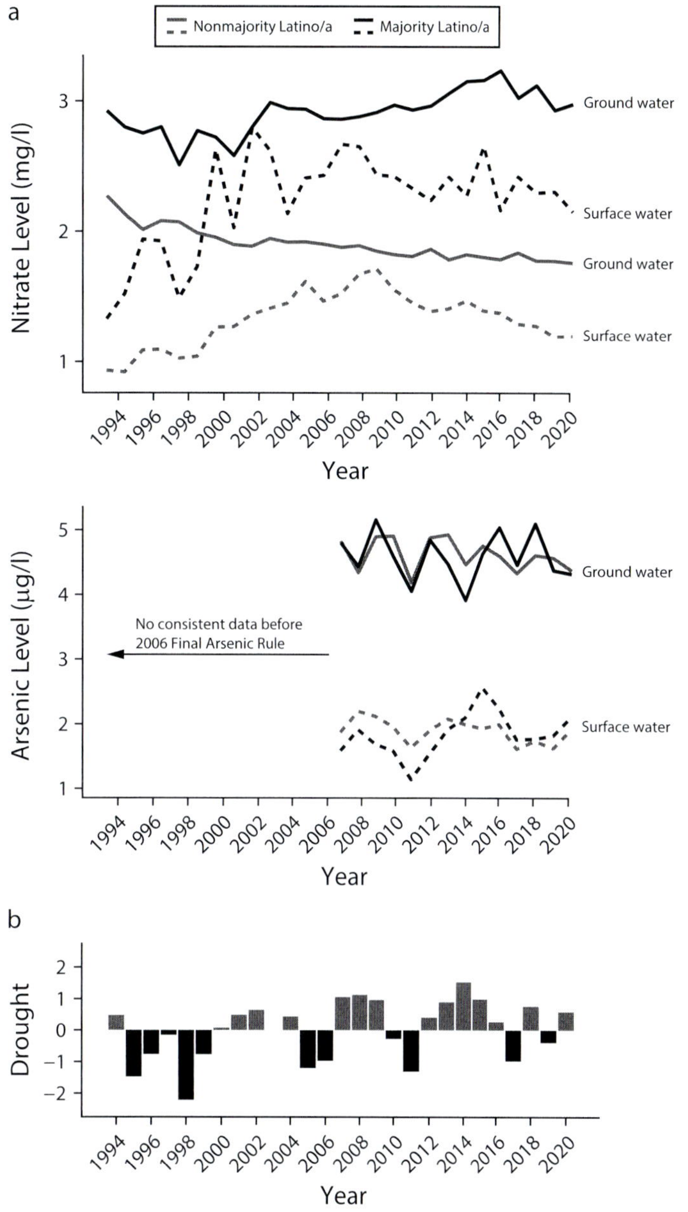

FIGURE 1— **Temporal Trends in (a) Contaminant Concentrations by Ethnic Composition of Community Water System (CWS) Service Area, and (b) Drought Index: California, 1994–2020**

Note. Trends start at 1994 for nitrate and 2007 for arsenic, a year after compliance monitoring (national primary drinking water regulations phase 2 and final arsenic rule) became operative for the contaminants. State-wide drought index determined by normalized Palmer Drought Severity Index. "Majority Latino/a" CWSs are characterized by serving a higher percentage of Latino/a population compared with any other racial or ethnic group. For a full-color version of this figure along with maps showing the spatial distribution of CWS service area boundaries serving majority Latino/a communities: California, 2020, and spatial distribution of drought index before (2011) and during (2014) the height of the historic 2012–2017 drought, see Appendix B (available as supplement to the online version of this article at https://www.ajph.org).

C represents nitrate (mg/l) or arsenic (µg/l) concentrations for sampling point *i* in CWS *w* in year *t*. *X* is one of the CWS subgroups: all; nonmajority Latino/a; more than 25%, 50%, and 75% majority Latino/a population; and low-income and agricultural regions. Sampling point fixed effects δ_i accounted for baseline concentrations associated with *i*. τ_w are CWS-specific linear year slopes that accounted for underlying long-term trends at the CWS level. D_{wt} is the normalized drought index experienced by CWS w in year t.

In Equation 1, β represents the average effect of a 1-unit increase on the normalized drought index on the contaminant concentration net of CWS time trends and sampling point baseline concentrations. In Equation 2, I included an interaction term with drought to indicate whether CWS w belongs to 1 of the sociodemographic subgroups, X, in year t. Now, β_0 represents the effect of drought but only for CWSs not in X (e.g., $1\{\%Latino/a > 50\} = 0$), and β_1 represents the mean difference in drought's effect for CWSs in group X (e.g., $1\{\%Latino/a > 50\} = 1$).

To address the potential issue of having multiple sampling points in each CWS, I used cluster-robust SEs at the CWS level. This method corrects for correlated error terms within each CWS and corrects the derived CIs.[30] I assigned weights to each CWS based on the total number of unique sampling points it had. Figure 2 plots $2 \times \hat{\beta}$ for all CWSs, $2 \times \hat{\beta}_0$ only for nonmajority Latino/a CWSs, and $2 \times (\hat{\beta}_0 + \hat{\beta}_1)$ for all other CWS subgroups, representing the effects of drought on DWN and DWA (I show the effects of a 2-unit increase in the normalized drought index because this scenario has occurred 3 times in the past 2 decades in California, specifically, during 2006–2007, 2011–2014, and 2017–2018), as illustrated in Figure 1. I conducted all statistical analyses in R version 4.2.2 (RStudio, Boston, MA).

RESULTS

Appendix B shows the distribution and service area boundaries of CWSs included in the analysis. The study sample covers 94% of Californians estimated to be served by a CWS and excludes the 3% of Californians who receive their drinking water from domestic wells, which are unregulated.[6] In this sample, there were 1732 (population served = 17.7 million) and 646 (population served = 17.1 million) CWSs serving nonmajority Latino/a and majority Latino/a communities, respectively. Table 1 shows that majority Latino/a CWSs are associated with more than twice the cropland area, 1.5 times the depth to groundwater table, and twice the mean nitrate concentrations than nonmajority Latino/a CWSs. Drought intensity, number of water sources, and arsenic concentration (Table 1) are relatively similar across these CWSs.

Figure 1 displays trends in DWN and DWA for majority Latino/a and all other CWSs. I show trends for surface water and groundwater drinking water samples separately because of significant differences in levels and trends. It is apparent that for both contaminants, pollutant concentrations have been more variable over the years for majority Latino/a CWSs than other CWSs. Groundwater-sourced DWN gradually increased from a low of 2.5 mg/l in 1998 to a peak of 3.1 mg/l in 2018 for majority Latino/s CWSs and decreased from 2.1 mg/l to 1.8 mg/l for nonmajority Latino/a CWSs over the same period. This widening exposure gap contrasts with recent articles documenting narrowing racial gaps in air pollution exposure.[31] Although DWN in surface sources decreased in the past decade for both groups, the mean DWN from surface sources for majority Latino/a CWSs (2.2 mg/l) was still significantly larger than that for other CWSs (1.2 mg/l) in 2020.

By contrast to DWN, DWA levels and trends for both CWS subgroups are similar. Figure 1 displays DWA trends starting from 2006, following the implementation of the Final Arsenic Rule, which introduced a systematic monitoring framework and lowered the arsenic MCL from 50 to 10 μg/l. DWA concentrations are notably higher for groundwater sources, averaging approximately 5 μg/l, compared with 2 μg/l for surface sources.

Drought conditions increase DWN concentrations only in CWSs with significant Latino/a populations, with the effect size increasing as the percentage of Latino/as served increases. Figure 2 shows that there are no drought effects for CWSs serving nonmajority Latino/a populations and low-income and agricultural regions. However, a 2-unit increase in the normalized drought index results in a 0.04 mg/l increase (2% of 2007 mean; 95% CI = 0.00, 0.08), 0.08 mg/l increase (4% of 2007 mean; 95% CI = 0.02, 0.14), and 0.16 mg/l increase (8% of 2007 mean; 95% CI = 0.02, 0.29) for CWSs with more than 25%, majority, and 75% Latino/a populations served, respectively. These results remain relatively unaffected and even more pronounced when using alternative fixed effects specifications (Appendix A, Tables B and C) and remain statistically significant even after controlling for a multitude of potential omitted variables, such as household income, surrounding groundwater depth, and measures of agricultural intensity (Appendix A, Figure B).

The uncovered nitrate drought effects vary across CWS characteristics. I reestimated the main analysis along 3 margins of interest: (1) source type, (2) system size, and (3) whether the CWS was managed by a local government or a private entity. Figure 3 shows that very small (< 500) and privately owned CWSs are driving the disproportionate drought effects and that DWN levels in surface sources are more

a

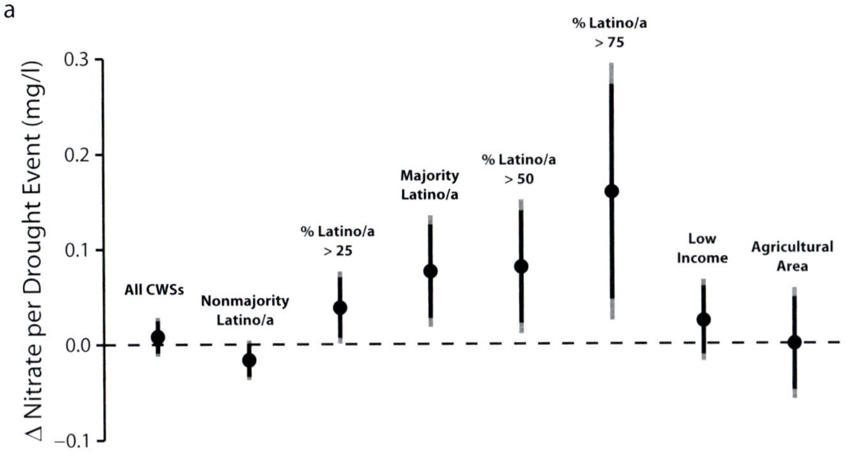

CWS subgroup	Nitrate drought response (mg/l)
All CWSs	0.01 (−0.01, 0.03)
Nonmajority Latino/a	−0.02 (−0.04, 0)
% Latino/a > 25	0.04 (0, 0.08)
Majority Latino/a	0.08 (0.02, 0.14)
% Latino/a > 50	0.08 (0.01, 0.15)
% Latino/a > 75	0.16 (0.02, 0.29)
Low Income	0.02 (−0.02, 0.07)
Agricultural Area	0 (−0.06, 0.06)

b

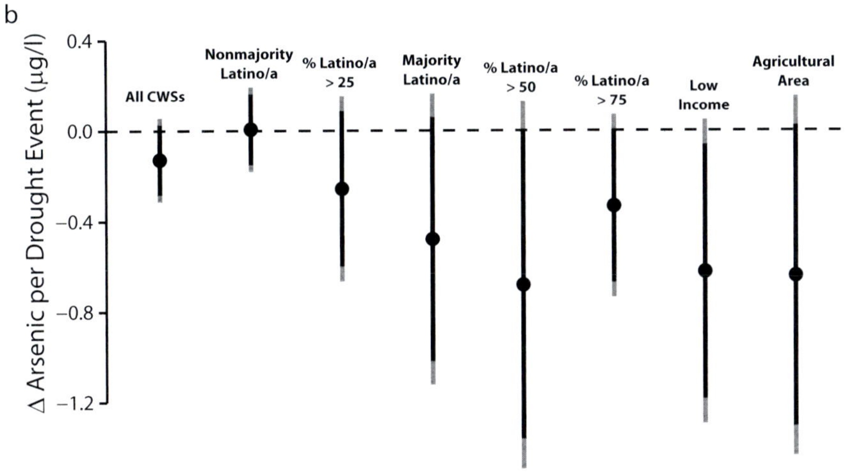

CWS subgroup	Arsenic drought response (µg/l)
All CWSs	−0.13 (−0.31, 0.06)
Nonmajority Latino/a	0.01 (−0.18, 0.19)
% Latino/a > 25	−0.26 (−0.67, 0.15)
Majority Latino/a	−0.48 (−1.12, 0.16)
% Latino/a > 50	−0.68 (−1.49, 0.13)
% Latino/a > 75	−0.33 (−0.74, 0.07)
Low Income	−0.62 (−1.3, 0.05)
Agricultural Area	−0.64 (−1.44, 0.15)

FIGURE 2— Heterogeneous Effects of Drought on Drinking Water Contaminants: California, 2007–2020

Note. CWS = community water system. Estimated effects of a 2-unit increase on the normalized drought index on nitrate (panel a) and arsenic (panel b) concentrations. Majority Latino/a CWSs are characterized by serving a higher percentage of Latino/a population compared with any other racial or ethnic group. Agricultural areas are defined as > 25% cropland in a 1 mi^2 radius. Gray and black lines represent 95% and 90% confidence intervals (CIs), respectively, calculated with SEs clustered at the CWS level. Point estimates are provided in accompanying tables, with 95% CIs in parentheses.

susceptible to increases during drought. Drought effects on DWN levels in surface sources (0.17 mg/l; 95% CI = 0.06, 0.28) are more than twice those in groundwater (0.07 mg/l; 95% CI = 0.01, 0.13) for majority Latino/a CWSs. Across all CWS features investigated, there is little to no drought effect on nitrate levels for nonmajority Latino/a CWSs.

Private CWSs include investor-owned utilities, water companies, and water associations; local government CWSs include municipalities, special districts, and cities (Table 1 shows a breakdown by type). For privately owned CWSs, drought increased DWN (0.12 mg/l; 95% CI = 0.04, 0.2) for majority Latino/a CWSs but had no significant effects for nonmajority Latino/a CWSs (−0.03; 95% CI = −0.06, 0.00). All CWSs subgroups managed by local governments had no significant drought effects on nitrate levels. Although majority Latino/a CWSs showed larger drought responses than other CWSs across all system sizes evaluated, the results are only significant and are most pronounced in very small CWSs (Figure 3). Across very small systems (< 500), nitrate concentrations increased by 0.11 mg/l (95% CI = 0.03, 0.2) for majority Latino/a CWSs only.

Drought conditions tend to decrease DWA, with effect sizes generally increasing with the percentage of Latino/a population served (Figure 2). Effect size ranged from −0.26 µg/l (7% of 2007 overall mean; 95% CI = −0.67, 0.15) to −0.68 µg/l (14% of 2007 overall mean; 95% CI = −1.49, 0.13) for CWSs serving more than 25% and 50% Latino/a populations, respectively.

a

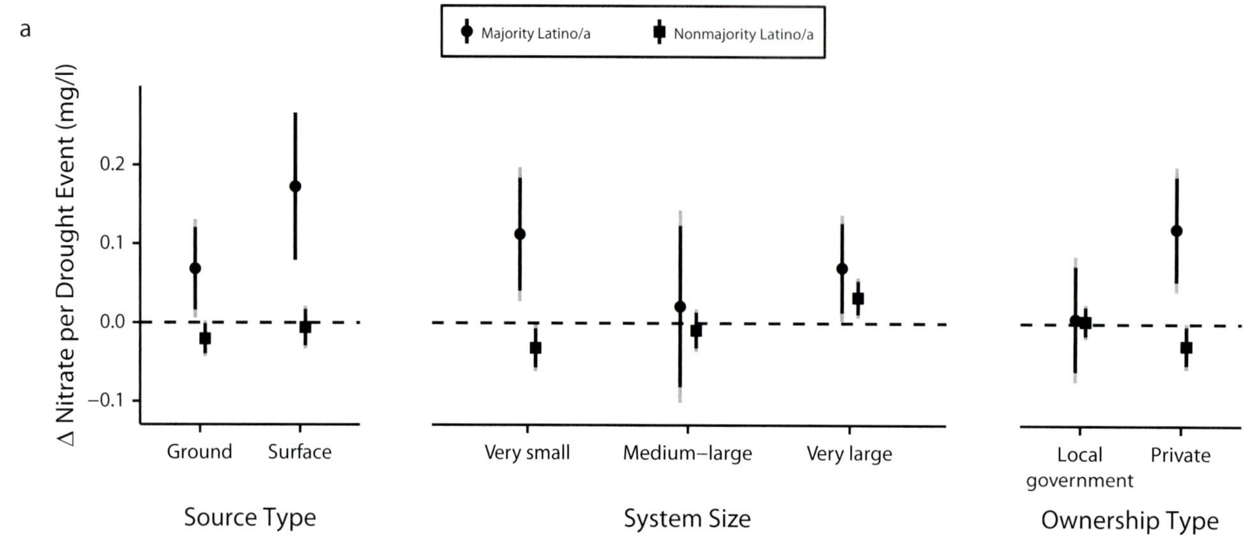

	Ground	Surface	Very small	Medium–large	Very large	Local government	Private
Majority Latino	0.07 (0.01, 0.13)	0.17 (0.06, 0.28)	0.11 (0.03, 0.2)	0.02 (−0.11, 0.14)	0.07 (0, 0.14)	0.01 (−0.07, 0.09)	0.12 (0.04, 0.2)
Nonmajority Latino	−0.02 (−0.04, 0)	−0.01 (−0.03, 0.02)	−0.03 (−0.06, 0)	−0.01 (−0.04, 0.02)	0.03 (0.01, 0.06)	0 (−0.02, 0.02)	−0.03 (−0.06, 0)

b

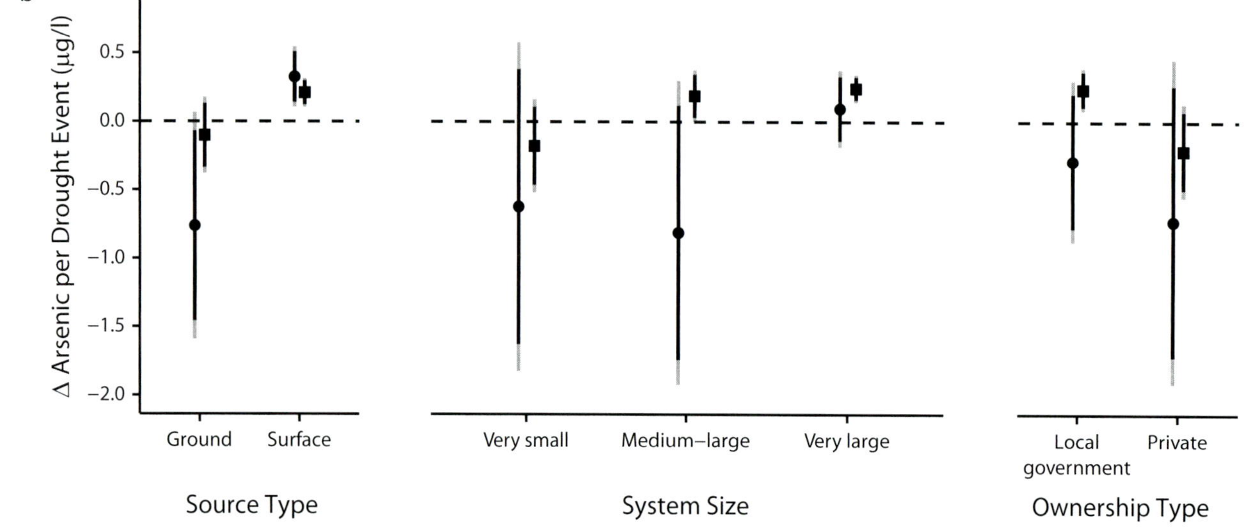

	Ground	Surface	Very small	Medium–large	Very large	Local government	Private
Majority Latino	−0.76 (−1.59, 0.07)	0.33 (0.11, 0.55)	−0.62 (−1.82, 0.58)	−0.81 (−1.92,0.3)	0.1 (−0.18, 0.38)	−0.29 (−0.88, 0.3)	−0.73 (−1.91, 0.46)
Nonmajority Latino	−0.1 (−0.38, 0.18)	0.21 (0.11, 0.32)	−0.18 (−0.52, 0.16)	0.19 (0, 0.38)	0.24 (0.14, 0.34)	0.24 (0.08, 0.39)	−0.21 (−0.55, 0.13)

FIGURE 3— Heterogeneous Effects of Drought on Drinking Water Contaminants Evaluated by Source Type and Community Water System (CWS) Characteristics: California, 2007–2020

Note. CI = confidence interval. Estimated effects of a 2-unit increase on the normalized drought index on nitrate (panel A) and arsenic (panel B) concentrations for nonmajority Latino/a (square) and majority Latino/a (circle) CWSs by water source type, CWS size, and ownership type. Gray and black lines represent 95% and 90% confidence intervals (CIs), respectively, calculated with SEs clustered at the CWS level. Point estimates are provided in accompanying tables, with 95% CIs in parentheses. "Majority Latino/a" CWSs are characterized by serving a higher percentage of Latino/a population compared with any other racial or ethnic group. CWS sizes were designated according to Environmental Protection Agency categories and adjusted by combining medium and large CWSs to form 3 groups of approximately equal size: very small (≤ 500 people), medium–large (500–10 000), and very large (> 10 000).

Although none of the estimated effects are statistically significant, the effect size is substantial. Figure 2 shows that CWSs serving low-income and agricultural regions experienced similar DWA level drought responses. Figure 3 shows that drought outcomes on DWA are heterogeneous by source type. Negative effects on DWA appear to be driven by groundwater sources.

Drought increased surface-sourced DWA for both groups (up to 0.33 µg/l; 95% CI = 0.11, 0.55 for majority Latino/a CWSs) and decreased groundwater DWA (–0.76 µg/l; 95% CI = −1.59, 0.07) only for majority Latino/a CWSs. Furthermore, there are significant and positive DWA drought effects for nonmajority Latino/a CWSs operated by local governments and those of medium to large sizes (Figure 3). These results reflect the surface water effect: more than 80% and 76% of surface sampling points in this subsample belong to local government and medium-large CWSs, respectively.

DISCUSSION

I found that Latino/a communities served by CWSs in California are vulnerable to increased nitrate concentrations in drinking water during drought conditions. These effects are especially magnified in surface-sourced drinking water and appear to be driven by very small and privately operated CWSs. The effect of drought on DWA concentrations is very variable. Drought increased overall arsenic concentrations in surface-sourced drinking water for both subgroups. Although statistically insignificant, drought decreased arsenic in groundwater-sourced drinking water for majority Latino/a communities.

A recent study revealed that drought increased nitrate prevalence by 3 to 5 times in public supply wells in the San Joaquin Valley, a major agricultural region in California, of which Latino/as form the largest ethnic group.[14] The authors found that drought leads to intensified agricultural groundwater pumping, which accelerates the downward flow of nitrate-contaminated water, elevating the nitrate concentration in water drawn by CWSs. Although the study corroborates the increased nitrate I observed in groundwater, it appears from my findings that surface water sources are more sensitive to drought conditions for both nitrate and arsenic in drinking water. This finding is concerning when we consider that although more CWSs (77%) are supplied by groundwater, more people (80%) are served by CWSs that use surface water as their primary source.

The differential effects I found suggest that CWSs serving Latino/a communities are not mitigating elevated nitrate concentrations during drought conditions, which exacerbates existing disparities. This may reflect a lack of treatment infrastructure, resource constraints, or other operational or technical differences. Although I focused on only arsenic and nitrate concentrations, these vulnerable CWSs may also be at increased risk for contamination from other sources (e.g., pesticides, waste disposal sites, and manufacturing plants) under stressors such as drought, floods, and other natural events. A recent review article highlighted a range of emerging drinking water contaminants of concern, including disinfection by-products and fracking-related substances, that disproportionately affect communities of color.[32]

Limitations

The limitations of this study ought to be discussed. First, because of the complex and highly localized nature of underground hydrogeological and geochemical processes, my study did not address the specific drought mechanisms causing the observed changes in arsenic and nitrate concentrations. Therefore, to what extent differential pumping, legacy contaminants, groundwater dynamics, and CWS mitigation are leading to the observed responses is a critical question for future research. Future studies could explore mechanisms behind the contrasting effects of drought on arsenic levels at surface and groundwater sampling points.

Second, data limitations may have contributed to uncertainty throughout the analysis. CWSs may have been assigned to the wrong sociodemographic subgroup because of uncertainties in the ACS data and water system service boundaries. Missing data from the water quality database, resulting from irregular sampling schedules or compliance issues, could have introduced bias to the parameter estimates. Although the main results did not change meaningfully in a sensitivity analysis in which I accounted explicitly for compounding errors from the ACS (Appendix A, Figure A), bias may still exist if there was ethnic/racial segregation in the census tracts that correlated with CWS service boundaries. I discuss these limitations in more detail in Appendix A, Section 1.5.

Public Health Implications

The severity of droughts in California has been greater in the past 2 decades than in the preceding century, and studies predict that the risk of severe drought will increase because of extremely warm conditions induced by anthropogenic climate change.[33] The disproportionate effects I have uncovered suggest that without significant investments in adaptive or mitigation capacity, future droughts may further widen drinking water disparities, putting already vulnerable communities at heightened risk.

These findings may help policymakers prioritize future research, funding, and technical assistance: (1) very small and private CWSs are driving the disproportionate drought effects experienced by Latino/a communities; (2) surface water sources are most reactive to drought conditions, and they serve a far greater proportion of the population; (3) arsenic decreased in groundwater-sourced drinking water only for Latino/a communities, which could reflect geochemical reactions resulting from concurrent increasing nitrate concentrations[16,17]; and (4) arsenic concentrations are heightened in surface-sourced drinking water during drought.

Although California earmarked more than $5.2 billion in its 2022 Water Supply Strategy to water systems for drought resilience, funding managers need to consider disparities and the potential rise of arsenic threats in funding and technical assistance allocation, especially under the state's 2021 Human Right to Water Law. Furthermore, statewide drinking water assistance programs such as the Safe and Affordable Drinking Water Fund should prioritize long-term and sustainable solutions over shorter-term ones, such as water deliveries, in the face of future drought-induced contaminant threats. AJPH

ABOUT THE AUTHORS

Sandy Sum is with the Bren School and the Department of Economics, University of California, Santa Barbara.

CORRESPONDENCE

Correspondence should be sent to Sandy Sum, Bren School of Environmental Science and Management, University of California, Santa Barbara, 3017 Bren Hall, Santa Barbara, CA 93106-5131 (e-mail: sandysum@ucsb.edu). Reprints can be ordered at https://www.ajph.org by clicking the "Reprints" link.

PUBLICATION INFORMATION

Full Citation: Sum S. Impact of droughts on served drinking water disparities in California, 2007–2020. *Am J Public Health*. 2024;114(9): 935–945.

Acceptance Date: June 10, 2024.

DOI: https://doi.org/10.2105/AJPH.2024.307758

ORCID iD:
Sandy Sum https://orcid.org/0000-0002-1681-9032

ACKNOWLEDGMENTS

This research was supported by the Central Coast Regional Equity Initiative from the University of California, Santa Barbara (UCSB) Blum Center and a graduate summer fellowship grant from the California Policy Lab.

I thank Tamma Carleton and Peiley Lau for their invaluable guidance and feedback. I also thank participants of the Columbia University Interdisciplinary PhD Workshop on Sustainable Development, the Workshop in Environmental Economics and Data Science, the UCSB 290 Environmental Economics seminar, and the Social Cost of Water Pollution Workshop for their helpful comments.

CONFLICTS OF INTEREST

The author has no conflicts of interest to declare.

HUMAN PARTICIPANT PROTECTION

This research did not involve human participants and therefore did not require institutional review board approval or exemption.

REFERENCES

1. Mullin M. The effects of drinking water service fragmentation on drought-related water security. *Science*. 2020;368(6488):274–277. https://doi.org/10.1126/science.aba7353
2. Pörtner H-O, Roberts DC, Tignor M, et al. Climate change 2022: impacts, adaptation and vulnerability. Available at: https://www.ipcc.ch/report/ar6/wg2. Accessed July 1, 2024.
3. Balazs C, Morello-Frosch R, Hubbard A, Ray I. Social disparities in nitrate-contaminated drinking water in California's San Joaquin Valley. *Environ Health Perspect*. 2011;119(9):1272–1278. https://doi.org/10.1289/ehp.1002878
4. Balazs CL, Morello-Frosch R, Hubbard AE, Ray I. Environmental justice implications of arsenic contamination in California's San Joaquin Valley: a cross-sectional, cluster-design examining exposure and compliance in community drinking water systems. *Environ Health*. 2012;11:84. https://doi.org/10.1186/1476-069X-11-84
5. Schaider LA, Swetschinski L, Campbell C, Rudel RA. Environmental justice and drinking water quality: are there socioeconomic disparities in nitrate levels in US drinking water? *Environ Health*. 2019;18:3. https://doi.org/10.1186/s12940-018-0442-6
6. Pace C, Balazs C, Bangia K, et al. Inequities in drinking water quality among domestic well communities and community water systems, California, 2011–2019. *Am J Public Health*. 2022; 112(1):88–97. https://doi.org/10.2105/AJPH.2021.306561
7. Balazs CL, Ray I. The Drinking Water Disparities Framework: On the origins and persistence of inequities in exposure. *Am J Public Health*. 2014;104(4):603–611. https://doi.org/10.2105/AJPH.2013.301664
8. Nigra AE, Chen Q, Chillrud SN, et al. Inequalities in public water arsenic concentrations in counties and community water systems across the United States, 2006–2011. *Environ Health Perspect*. 2020;128(12):127001. https://doi.org/10.1289/EHP7313
9. Foster SA, Pennino MJ, Compton JE, Leibowitz SG, Kile ML. Arsenic drinking water violations decreased across the United States following revision of the maximum contaminant level. *Environ Sci Technol*. 2019;53(19):11478–11485. https://doi.org/10.1021/acs.est.9b02358
10. Ward MH, Jones R, Brender J, et al. Drinking water nitrate and human health: an updated review. *Int J Environ Res Public Health*. 2018; 15(7):1557. https://doi.org/10.3390/ijerph15071557
11. Naujokas MF, Anderson B, Ahsan H, et al. The broad scope of health effects from chronic arsenic exposure: update on a worldwide public health problem. *Environ Health Perspect*. 2013; 121(3):295–302. https://doi.org/10.1289/ehp.1205875
12. Essien EE, Said Abasse K, Côté A, et al. Drinking-water nitrate and cancer risk: a systematic review and meta-analysis. *Arch Environ Occup Health*. 2022;77(1):51–67. https://doi.org/10.1080/19338244.2020.1842313
13. Thaw M, GebreEgziabher M, Villafañe-Pagán JY, Jasechko S. Modern groundwater reaches deeper depths in heavily pumped aquifer systems. *Nat Commun*. 2022;13(1):1–9. https://doi.org/10.1038/s41467-022-32954-1
14. Levy ZF, Jurgens BC, Burow KR, et al. Critical aquifer overdraft accelerates degradation of groundwater quality in California's Central Valley during drought. *Geophys Res Lett*. 2021;48(17): e2021GL094398. https://doi.org/10.1029/2021GL094398
15. Smith R, Knight R, Fendorf S. Overpumping leads to California groundwater arsenic threat. *Nat Commun*. 2018;9(1):1–6. https://doi.org/10.1038/s41467-018-04475-3
16. Smith RL, Kent DB, Repert DA, Böhlke JK. Anoxic nitrate reduction coupled with iron oxidation and attenuation of dissolved arsenic and phosphate in a sand and gravel aquifer. *Geochim Cosmochim Acta*. 2017;196:102–120. https://doi.org/10.1016/j.gca.2016.09.025
17. Haugen EA, Jurgens BC, Arroyo-Lopez JA, Bennett GL. Groundwater development leads to decreasing arsenic concentrations in the San Joaquin

Valley, California. *Sci Total Environ*. 2021;771:145223. https://doi.org/10.1016/j.scitotenv.2021.145223

18. Welch AH, Lico MS, Hughes JL. Arsenic in ground water of the Western United States. *Groundwater*. 1988;26(3):333–347. https://doi.org/10.1111/j.1745-6584.1988.tb00397.x
19. Müller V, Chavez-Capilla T, Feldmann J, Mestrot A. Increasing temperature and flooding enhance arsenic release and biotransformations in Swiss soils. *Sci Total Environ*. 2022;838(pt 1):156049. https://doi.org/10.1016/j.scitotenv.2022.156049
20. State of California. Annual compliance report data-set 2019. Available at: https://www.waterboards.ca.gov/drinking_water/certlic/drinkingwater/docs/acr_2019_final.pdf. Accessed February 27, 2024.
21. Harter T, Lund JR, Darby J, et al. Addressing nitrate in California's drinking water with a focus on Tulare Lake Basin and Salinas Valley groundwater. 2012. Available at: https://ucanr.edu/sites/groundwaternitrate/files/138956.pdf. Accessed February 27, 2024.
22. California Department of Water Resources. Drinking water treatment and distribution 2016. Available at: https://water.ca.gov/-/media/DWR-Website/Web-Pages/Programs/California-Water-Plan/Docs/RMS/2016/14_Drinking_Water_Treatment_Distribution_July2016.pdf. Accessed February 27, 2024.
23. Blaisdell J, Turyk ME, Almberg KS, Jones RM, Stayner LT. Prenatal exposure to nitrate in drinking water and the risk of congenital anomalies. *Environ Res*. 2019;176:108553. [Erratum in: *Environ Res*. 2020;186:109269. https://doi.org/10.1016/j.envres.2020.109269]. https://doi.org/10.1016/j.envres.2019.108553
24. García-Esquinas E, Pollán M, Umans JG, et al. Arsenic exposure and cancer mortality in a US-based prospective cohort: the Strong Heart Study. *Cancer Epidemiol Biomarkers Prev*. 2013;22(11):1944–1953. https://doi.org/10.1158/1055-9965.EPI-13-0234-T
25. Saint-Jacques N, Parker L, Brown P, Dummer TJB. Arsenic in drinking water and urinary tract cancers: a systematic review of 30 years of epidemiological evidence. *Environ Health*. 2014;13:44. https://doi.org/10.1186/1476-069X-13-44
26. Holtby CE, Guernsey J, Allen A, VanLeeuwen J, Allen V, Gordon R. A population-based case–control study of drinking-water nitrate and congenital anomalies using geographic information systems (GIS) to develop individual-level exposure estimates. *Int J Environ Res Public Health*. 2014;11(2):1803–1823. https://doi.org/10.3390/ijerph110201803
27. Laura A, Komal B, Laurel P, et al. CalEnviroScreen 4.0 2021. Available at: https://oehha.ca.gov/media/downloads/calenviroscreen/report/calenviroscreen40reportf2021.pdf. Accessed February 27, 2024.
28. CA Division of Drinking Water. California drinking water system area boundaries 2022. Available at: https://gis.data.ca.gov/datasets/waterboards::california-drinking-water-system-area-boundaries/about. Accessed June 2, 2022.
29. Abatzoglou JT. Development of gridded surface meteorological data for ecological applications and modelling. *Int J Climatol*. 2013;33(1):121–131. https://doi.org/10.1002/joc.3413
30. Abadie A, Athey S, Imbens GW, Wooldridge JM. When should you adjust standard errors for clustering? *Q J Econ*. 2022;138(1):1–35. https://doi.org/10.1093/qje/qjac038
31. Hernandez-Cortes D, Meng KC. Do environmental markets cause environmental injustice? Evidence from California's carbon market. *J Public Econ*. 2023;217:104786. https://doi.org/10.1016/j.jpubeco.2022.104786
32. Levin R, Villanueva CM, Beene D, et al. US drinking water quality: exposure risk profiles for seven legacy and emerging contaminants. *J Expo Sci Environ Epidemiol*. 2024;34(1):3–22. https://doi.org/10.1038/s41370-023-00597-z
33. Diffenbaugh NS, Swain DL, Touma D. Anthropogenic warming has increased drought risk in California. *Proc Natl Acad Sci U S A*. 2015;112(13):3931–3936. https://doi.org/10.1073/pnas.1422385112

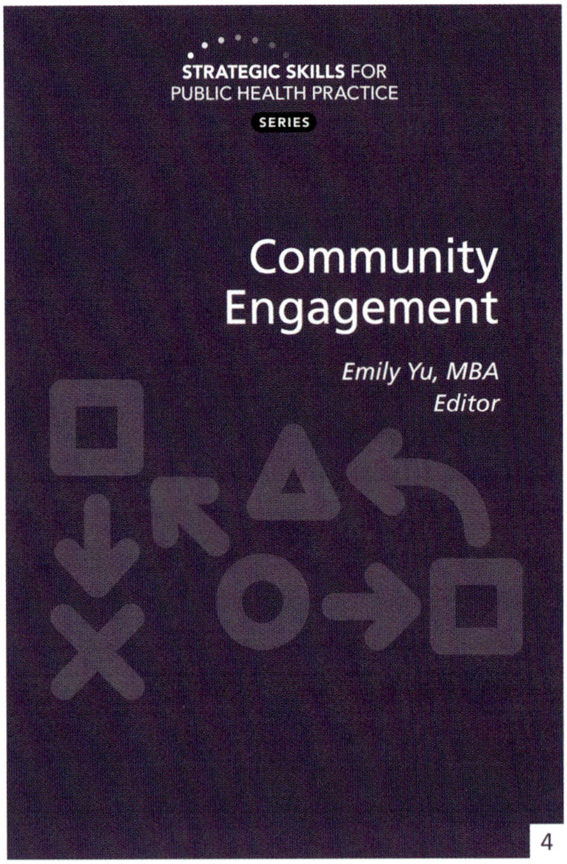

978-087553-3308, 108 PP, DIGITAL & SOFTCOVER

Community Engagement

Edited by Emily Yu, MBA

Community Engagement is the first book to be published from our new *Strategic Skills for Public Health Practice* series. This book brings the concept of community engagement to life through first-person stories, real-world examples and valuable insights from leaders across sectors. Curated specifically for public health practitioners and those interested in supporting community health, the book's chapters, guidance, and perspectives from the field will enhance readers' understanding of community-centered design and provide the tools to support organizational practices that drive better health for all.

APHABOOKSTORE.ORG

APHA PRESS

AN IMPRINT OF AMERICAN PUBLIC HEALTH ASSOCIATION

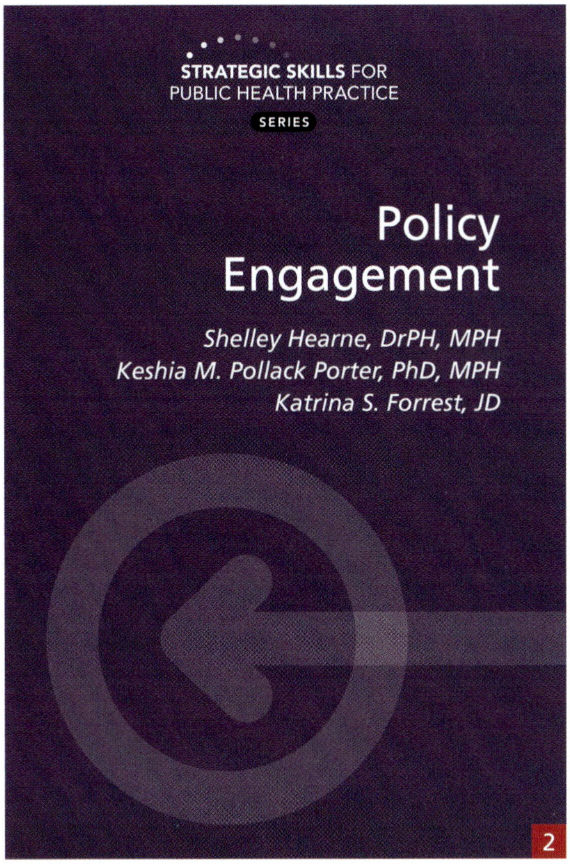

978-087553-3384, 200 PP., 2023
DIGITAL AND SOFTCOVER

Policy Engagement

By Shelley Hearne, DrPH,
Keshia M. Pollack Porter, PhD,
and Katrina S. Forrest, JD

Policy Engagement is a field guide for public health practitioners (from government workers to nonprofit leaders) on engaging with policymakers to create a healthier, more equitable world. This easy-to-read introduction to policy advocacy and decision-making offers a toolkit of concrete, practical, and insightful strategies for informing and influencing policymakers.

Part of the Strategic Skills for Public Health Practice series, *Policy Engagement* demystifies policymaking to help public health professionals become engaged, energized, and effective advocates for policies that drive better health.

APHABOOKSTORE.ORG

APHA PRESS

Standard Methods for the Examination of Dairy Products, 18th edition

Edited by Jeffrey L. Kornacki, PhD, Elliot T. Ryser, PhD, and Cynthia M. Mangione; Managing Editor: H. Michael Wehr, PhD

Standard Methods for the Examination of Dairy Products is a widely-recognized source of methods to assess the safety and quality of dairy products. It is an overview of microbiological, chemical and physical methods for analyzing milk and dairy products, designed for use by regulatory, industry and commercial laboratories. As with earlier editions, the 18th edition of Standard Methods for the Examination of Dairy Products:

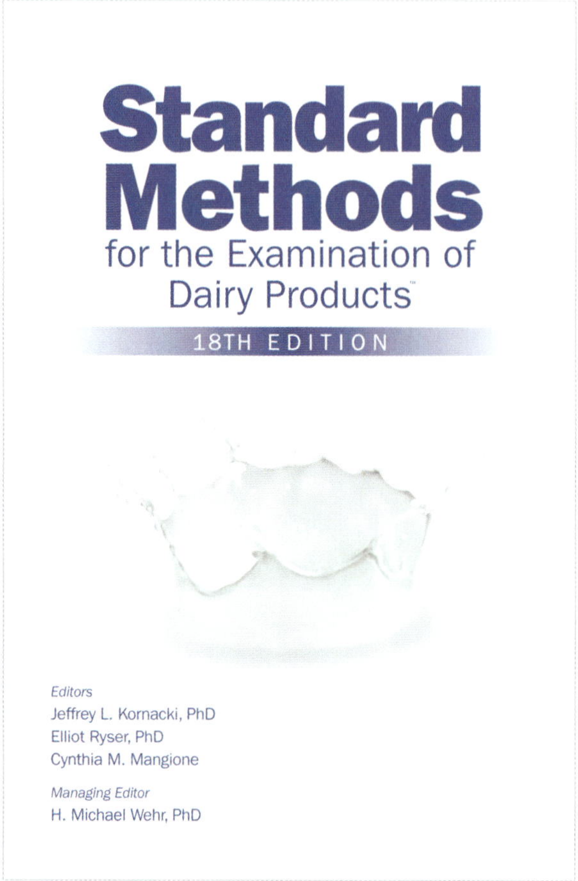

9780-887553-3421, SOFTCOVER, 1144 PP, 2024

- Highlights test methods that are a critical component of both government and industry analytical programs.
- Provides methods that foster uniformity in the testing of milk and milk programs.

This new 18th Edition of SMEDP updates and expands upon earlier editions of this authoritative reference, including:

- Comprehensive revision to chapters on antibiotic drug residues, pathogens, chemical and physical methods, and methods for heat process verification.
- Updates on both automated, and molecular-based methods.

APHABOOKSTORE.ORG

APHA PRESS

AN IMPRINT OF AMERICAN PUBLIC HEALTH ASSOCIATION

APHA 2024

ANNUAL MEETING & EXPO

Minneapolis | Oct. 27-30

Rebuilding Trust in Public Health and Science

CAN'T MISS EVENTS

WOMEN'S LEADERSHIP INSTITUTE*
Saturday, Oct. 26 | 9 a.m.-2:30 p.m.

OPENING SESSION
Rebuilding Trust In Public Health & Science
Sunday, Oct. 27 | 11 a.m -12:30 p.m.

LIVE TAPING OF THE AMERICA DISSECTED PODCAST
Trauma, Trust and Why We Still Haven't Processed the Pandemic with Professor Eric Klinenberg
Sunday, Oct. 27 | 4:30 p.m.-6 p.m.
Host: Abdul El Sayed

APHA AWARDS CEREMONY AND LUNCHEON*
Monday, Oct. 28 | 12:30-2 p.m.

MONDAY GENERAL SESSION
Improving the Public's Health: Looking Forward
Monday, Oct. 28 | 4:30-6 p.m.

CLOSING SESSION
APHA 2025: Making the Public's Health A Top Priority
Wednesday, Oct. 30 | 2:30-4 p.m.

*event will require a purchased ticket to attend

Explore the full schedule, presenters and sessions at **APHA.ORG/PROGRAM.**

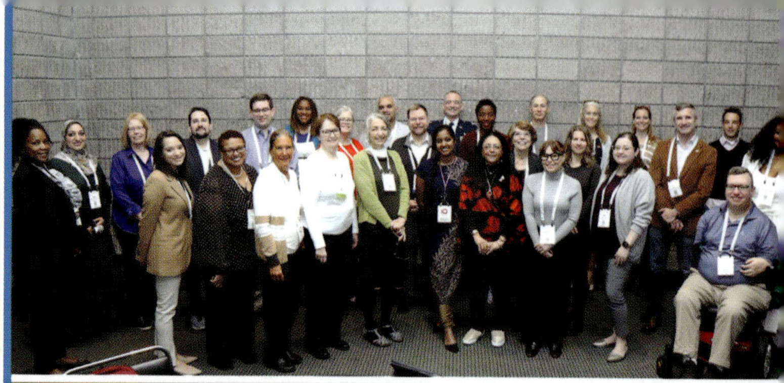

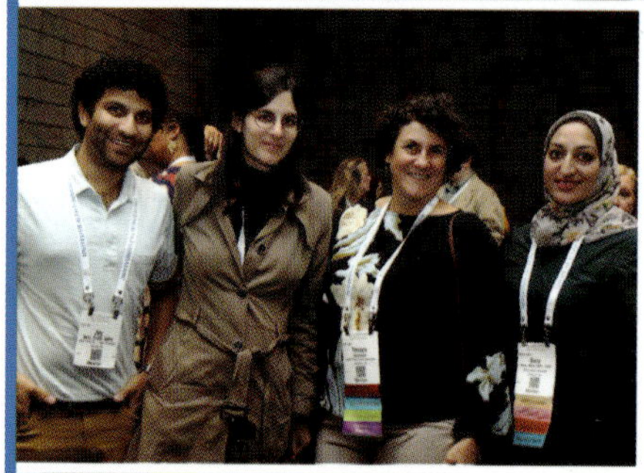

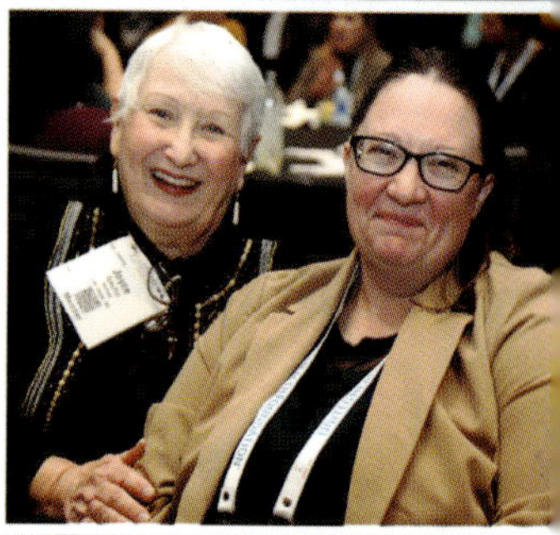

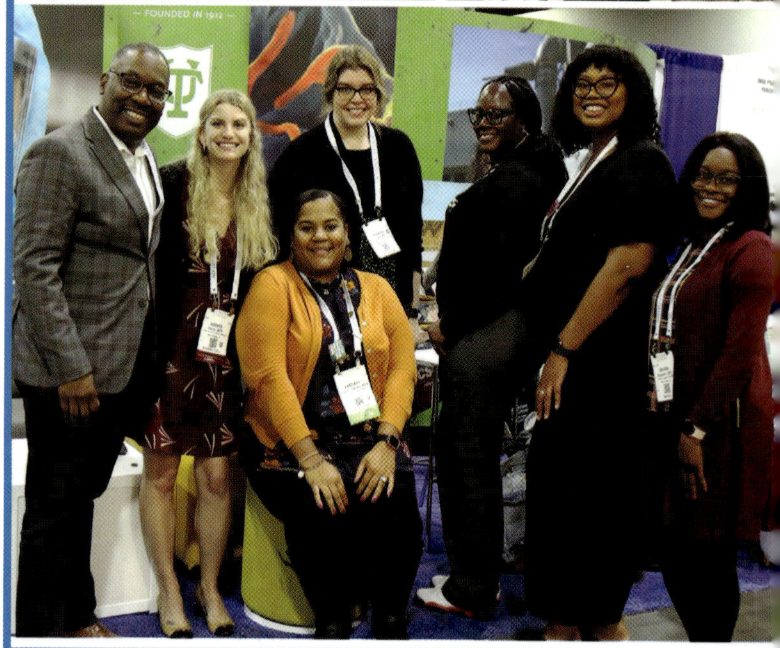

REGISTER NOW

before prices increase on Sept.16!

APHA.org/AnnualMeeting

CAN'T TRAVEL?

We're hosting a digital version of APHA 2024 from Oct. 26-30. This will include on-demand content and access to oral session presentation recordings from the in-person meeting. All recordings are available to you until Dec. 31, 2024.